$34.99
+tax

[inspired lives]

D1469623

[the best of real life yoga from ascent magazine]

inspired lives

edited by Clea McDougall

timeless books 2005

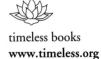

timeless books
www.timeless.org

© 2005 timeless books

In Canada:
Box 9, Kootenay Bay, BC
V0B 1X0
contact@timeless.org
(800) 661-8711

In the United States:
P.O. Box 3543, Spokane, WA   99220-3543
info@timeless.org
(800) 251-9273

Cover photograph by Chloe Dulude
Design by Todd Stewart   www.breeree.com

This edition is printed in Canada on 100% post-consumer waste, recycled acid-free paper.

Library and Archives Canada Cataloguing in Publication

   Inspired lives : the best of real life yoga from ascent
magazine / edited by Clea McDougall.

ISBN 1-932018-11-5

   1. Yoga. I. McDougall, Clea II. Title: Ascent (Kootenay Bay, B.C.).

B132.Y6I57 2005   181'.45   C2005-904139-0

timeless books and *ascent* magazine gratefully acknowledge the support of the Yasodhara Ashram Society, The Friends of Radha Foundation, the Association for the Development of Human Potential and the many individuals who have contributed to sustaining these publishing projects.

table of contents

Part Three: Reflection / Encounters with Self

preface: ascension

*a*scent had its name before I ever came along as editor in 1999. It had been around for thirty years at that point, as a small community newsletter for Yasodhara Ashram in British Columbia. We kept the name, but expanded into a full-sized, international magazine. I have always harboured a secret pleasure for the title of the magazine, because the first jazz record I ever bought, and subsequently fell in love with, was *Ascension* by John Coltrane.

I actually had no idea what the record would be like at the time I bought it. Not really a place for an eighteen year old to start her jazz education. Or maybe it was *the* place. Recorded in 1965, it is known as the turning point of Coltrane's career. *Ascension* marked his shift from traditional chord change structured jazz to free jazz. It is a session of Coltrane and his musicians letting go in one of their first experimentations of pure ecstatic playing. *Ascension* is said to be his step to liberty.

I didn't know any of that. I was just taken in by the story of the *Ascension* session on the back of the record. One of the musicians, Marion Brown, described the session as "wildly exciting. We did two takes and they both had that kind of thing in them that makes people scream. The people who were in the studio *were* screaming. I don't know how the engineers kept the screams off the record."

"This is a guaranteed soul rinsing," wrote A.B. Spellman. "There is impact and release, communion and response; the emphasis is on the unmentionable, on what I call the Marvelous. It is not intended that *Ascension* will be background music for polite dinner conversation."

And it's not an easy record to listen to. But if you let yourself be pulled into the seeming chaos of it, you know these people are in touch with something beyond themselves. They were totally and absolutely inspired.

I became a lover of avant jazz after that, especially Coltrane's later work. I loved the spirit of it, the willingness to explore and the desire to find a divine expression through music.

So, yes, *ascent* pleased me. Not that we were doing anything comparable to free jazz, but the idea of "ascension" itself was an inspiration. We wanted yoga to go beyond doctrine or a system of stretches, and be about the way we live, how we encounter life. I wanted to find that, and celebrate the yogis, the people who were trying to live consciously, humbly, embracing everything that came to them, exploring and redefining spiritual life. It was this largeness that we aimed for, this stepping off into liberty.

And a little like the record, I really had no idea what I was getting into when I took the job of editor at *ascent* magazine. It definitely wasn't what I expected. I couldn't have predicted the events of the years ahead, how *ascent* would change me, that the magazine would turn into what it is today, or how it could inspire such a fierce loyalty in its readers. We just had a vision of how to explore yoga, what it could look like, how it could be lived, practised and loved.

We found others who were equally dedicated to this endeavour; they became the voices and faces of the magazine. The best of what came out of this collaboration is assembled in this book.

As *Inspired Lives* is being published, *ascent* is well into its seventh year and continues its publishing adventures. The essays and interviews in this book have been collected from 1999–2004, the first six years of *ascent*'s life (also the approximate time that I was editor. I left the magazine after the fall issue 2004: Liberation!). The pieces are a collection that in my view represents the essence of *ascent*. The stories are about the diverse lives of yogis, Buddhists, Christians, musicians, artists and political activists. Typical of *ascent*, some of these lives may stretch the limit of what we, at first glance, recognize as yoga. However, I feel that this is yoga in its most truthful and relevant sense: the search for how we can live a spiritual life in our modern world.

Working on the book, I was touched by the collective honesty here. Even though I have read these articles innumerable times and worked closely with the authors over the years, each essay seemed fresh and there were numerous moments when I was moved to tears. There is just something incredibly sincere about the voices of *ascent*, what they speak to, their acceptance of the joys and difficulties in being human. I think the special gift that *ascent* has is that it provides a forum for this work of yoga, the real life work.

One contributor recently wrote to me: "One of the things I like about *ascent* is that the 'happy-happy' and health-oriented spirituality so much in vogue is countered by a mature 'real world' spirituality, that crosses every boundary and border and belief system."

The thing about true inspiration is that it isn't all happiness and prettiness and ease. It isn't the cosmetic niceness that we tend to desire in the Western world. Just like the *Ascension* album, which isn't necessarily easy to listen to, inspiration doesn't always look the way we want it to look. It can be chaotic and painful and not very pretty at all. But often out of that pain and mess comes the beautiful, real stuff of life.

This book is dedicated to the people who sincerely want to live a spiritual life, those who are asking: Where do we find yoga, how do we live it, how do we get inspired, inspire ourselves, inspire others? What is the step we can take to find liberation?

These are questions I ask myself every day. Knowing there are others out there, such as all these authors and subjects and stories and lives well lived, knowing they too are on this path, asking these questions, has lent much needed inspiration.

Clea McDougall
Barcelona, June 2005

foreword: be inspired

my grandfather, Tirumalai Krishnamacharya, was over 100 years old when he died. The list of his accomplishments is long. I know them by heart now – diplomas and honours from the best universities in India, eight years of grueling study with his master in the Himalayas, teacher to kings, writer of articles and books and poetry, healer of thousands, the yogi, many would agree, who revived the dying art of yoga in the early twentieth century.

How did he manage to do all of this, as well as raise a family and live a fulfilling life?

Inspiration.

What is it, this inspiration? We throw the word around a lot, but do we always know what we are talking about when we use it? Can you see inspiration? Can you hold it in your hand? What colour is it? What shape? How big or small? You think of a moment in time when you said to yourself or someone else, "I was inspired to do this or that…" and then you try to trace this inspiration back to its source, but what you find is that at some point, you lose the trail, the tracks fade and there is only a sense of wonder and feelings half-remembered – of calm, clarity and focused energy.

I was fourteen years old when my grandfather died. I did not know about his accomplishments then. I knew him through experience, through proximity. Through play and laughter and the classroom, where he taught me and other children yoga poses, weaving them into stories, enchanting us and exciting us. And then he would gift each of us with one of his favourite confections made of sugar and almonds before sending us home. He loved me, played with me, taught me, shared with me. These are the things I knew about him first.

When I was nine, he fell and broke his hips. I remember I was worried that

17

he would not be able to play with me anymore. Doctors came at the beginning, but he sent them away. He told everyone he would heal himself through his yoga. He was ninety-six years old. Within a few months, he was able to take some small steps. He was never as agile as he was before the fall, but he walked. And he taught. And we played. And he wrote the two books that are considered his finest works. Right up until his death, he lived his life. For these reasons, I loved him. He inspired me. He still does.

My sister got married last month and moved away from our home to live with her husband in Detroit. Her traditional Indian wedding, which lasted three days, took place only two weeks after we had returned from a series of yoga conferences that whisked us through ten countries in eight weeks. I was still not fully recovered from the trip and the wedding when the emotional impact of my sister's departure began to manifest itself in our household. On top of this, twenty-three of my students are in Chennai for our semi-annual studies, and I am needed in the classroom from dawn until dusk. I am tired and my two-year-old daughter wants to play with me as soon as I get home in the evening. I would like to play, too, but I also want some sleep, and my parents are sad from missing my sister, so I want to be close to them and make them happy again. I was feeling so tired that I could not bring myself to sit down and write this foreword. The thing I was to write about – inspiration – was the thing I was having trouble finding.

Inspiration returned, though, as it always does, invoked by my strong memories of my grandfather. While teaching my students, I had to give an example of someone who never gave up – who was always inspired. I shared memories of my grandfather, how he lived his life never losing faith, committed to yoga and his practice, to healing, to his family and his God. I shared some of his poems. By the end of class, I felt better. When I returned home that night, I sat down and began to write.

There are reminders of him all around me – some obvious, such as pictures, the words he wrote, his ring on my finger, the sanctuary in the garden where we keep his *padukas*, his sandals that in Indian tradition symbolize the teachings. Other reminders are not so obvious. Memories. Feelings. It is to memory and feeling that I turn the most when I need his inspiration. Things mean little without the memories that give them life. It is the feelings he evoked in me that help me connect with the source of inspiration.

But even without these memories of my grandfather, without his example,

I can connect with the source of inspiration, because it exists inside of me, as it does in every person. We only have to find a way to access it. My memories of my grandfather are one portal for me. My yoga practice is another source of inspiration.

A good yoga practice can inspire us; it can help us to connect to the source of inspiration within us by clearing the cluttered mind. My most creative moments are when my mind is quiet, after I have done my practice, after I have done my chanting, after I have done my meditation, or even after teaching a class.

At the same time, by clearing the mind yoga also makes us sensitive to the infinite beauty of the world outside of us. Like us, every element of this world contains the source of inspiration like a hidden seed. If we are sensitive, if the mind is uncluttered, receptive and pure, we perceive the world around us with clear eyes and an open heart, and the most ordinary things inspire us. They remind us that what we think we cannot find – the ability to trust or to act unselfishly, or even the will to face another day when life seems hopeless – these abilities exist in abundance all around us. We tend to think that we must "find" inspiration, as if it were something lost or far away and separate from us, but it is right here, where we are, available to us at any moment.

And so, I do my yoga practice, just as my grandfather did his every day of his life for almost 100 years. It inspired him to share yoga with everyone who would listen, so that they, too, could be inspired and live life with a free and open heart. Inspiration is like a flame; it wants to be shared, it wants to light a spark in every person it touches.

For six years now, *ascent*, with uncommon eloquence and creativity, has been exploring how the practice of yoga affects the way we see the world and live our life, how it brings us closer to what we are seeking – to the unchanging source of inspiration. Each journey in this book is unique, just as each one of us is unique, but the search is universal and the source belongs to all of us.

Be Inspired.

Kausthub Desikachar
Chennai, India, July 2005

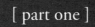

[part one]

engagement / encounters with community

Part of *ascent's* passion is being able to present an alternative to popular yoga. One of the ways the magazine does this is by standing up for how yoga takes action in our lives and in our world. To this aim *ascent* features stories of what is now being called spiritual activism or engaged spirituality. Not only are these activists huge inspirations for us, but by emphasizing their stories we can hopefully support social and individual evolution, and become more aware of the ever evolving forms of serious spiritual practice.

As Georg Feuerstein says in his interview with Swami Gopalananda, the future of yoga "will be a yoga that will be socially and politically engaged because that's part of our existence. Our job will be much more how to integrate all the different aspects and levels of our being, how to live in the world in a spiritual way."

Here are encounters with community, encounters calling on compassion, selflessness and devotion.

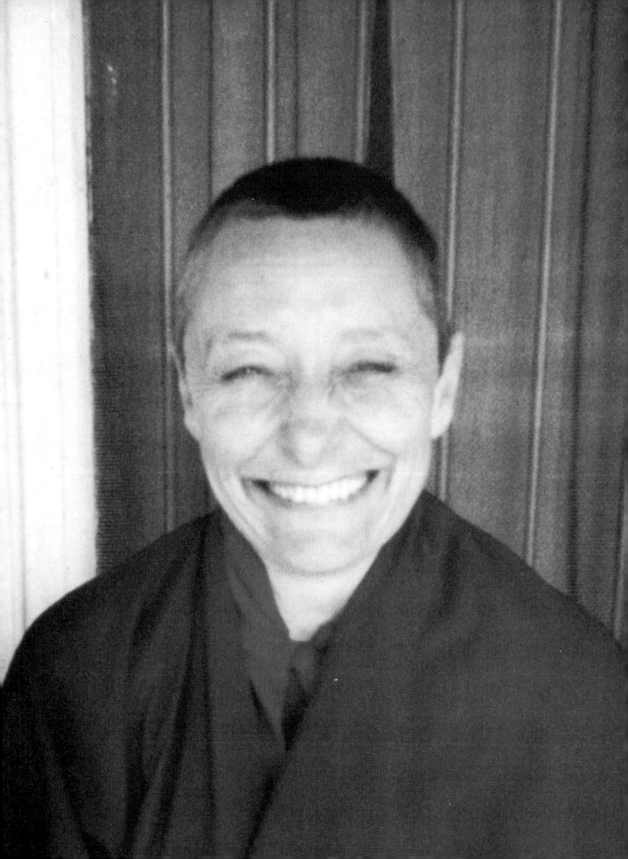

First published in Issue 4, Leadership, Winter 1999

tenzin palmo is watering the nuns

restoring a female lineage

[Tenzin Palmo interviewed by Lesley Marian Neilson]

t enzin Palmo is a Buddhist nun who is becoming known around the world as the Englishwoman who spent twelve years in a cave, high in the Himalayas. She is also a Buddhist who has vowed to attain enlightenment in a woman's body, challenging the institutionalized belief that only the male form can reach Liberation. She now travels internationally giving talks wherever she is invited to speak, in order to raise funds to build a nunnery in northern India. She is a dynamic incarnation of the emerging and powerful feminine principle in Buddhism.

Tenzin Palmo's voice is clear and sweet as she talks to me over the phone. It took two attempts to get a line between this small town in the Kootenays, British Columbia, and Dharamsala, India, where she is spending a few weeks before returning to Kangra to look at land to purchase, on which she will build the nunnery. It is to be known as Dongyu Gatsal Ling, which means Delightful Grove of the True Lineage. Tenzin Palmo has been working since 1993 to finance the

photo by Monica Joyce

project, and we begin our conversation with her talking about the stage the project has reached:

Tenzin Palmo   What we are doing is starting a nunnery which will be especially for girls from the Himalayan border region, including Ladakh, Bhutan, Lahul. These are areas where there is a long tradition of Buddhism, but where, although they have monks and nuns both, the nuns have really not been given any opportunity for study or for more deep practice. I lived for many years in one of these Himalayan regions and I saw for myself that essentially the nuns are just servants either to their family or to the monks. And it's a pity because these girls are very bright, very intelligent. As soon as they're given an opportunity to study and to practise, then it's like they're tight little buds which, if they're given enough sunshine and rain and fertilizer, just open up and blossom. One is seeing that now. Particularly from my tradition we want to encourage that. Because there is nothing at the moment for these nuns.

Lesley Marian Neilson   Was it your experience in the monasteries when you came over to India that really opened your eyes to the inequalities between the nuns and monks?

TP   Yes, well, it's just part of the social fabric. It was not considered necessary for women to be educated, or for nuns to follow the same kind of educational program as the monks. Because nobody ever had done that, everybody accepted that's the way it is. Nowadays, more and more, they are starting schools for nuns, where nuns can carry on the same kind of educational curriculum as the monks, and the nuns are absolutely flourishing. They are doing so well, because they don't just take it for granted. If someone does show an interest in them, if people do think that the nuns have potential, then, as I say, they absolutely flower, they really blossom. It's wonderful to see it; it's terribly encouraging.

LMN   What are the challenges you face in building a monastery for women?

TP   One of the problems is finding adequate teachers. In my particular tradition there are not that many qualified teachers of philosophy. And because they will be teaching nuns, one has to be very careful. Inviting young monks in to teach is sort of precarious, and older monks might feel that there's not much status in teaching nuns. They may get teased by other monks. They probably would feel quite lonely because they won't have that kind of monastic community which they're used to. Obviously they can't socialize very much with the nuns. And so this I see is going to be a challenge, finding good teachers.

In the future there will actually be nuns who will be qualified to teach. There are some monasteries which are now doing a full-scale educational program for the nuns, and some nuns have been in that already for some years. So eventually they will be qualified and then they could be invited to come and teach. That would be ideal. Not only would there then not be the problem of monks and nuns mixing, but also they would be a role model for the younger nuns themselves – instead of always thinking it's the monks who have the authority and the learning, and we're just women.

LMN   Do you have a sense of why these changes are happening now? What's allowing a tradition, which for thousands of years hasn't had much of a place for women, to open up?

TP   I think, first of all, there's a whole global interest in women. That's the outer cause. One of the inner causes is that nowadays the monasteries for the monks are pretty well established. Previously, when the Tibetans came out as refugees, their first aim was to get themselves re-established, to rebuild the monasteries, to see that everything didn't die out. There was a kind of desperation. That now has been taken care of. There are dozens if not hundreds of monasteries, thousands of monks – the tradition is not in danger of dying out. That's one thing. Now they have the space to begin to realize there is a whole other side to Buddhism; there is a whole female side.

The other thing is that through the years there have been a number of Western nuns who have become very well educated, often already with MAs in Buddhist philosophy from Western universities, who have come and studied, for example at the dialectic school in Dharamsala, and who have done extremely well. That has also opened up the eyes of the establishment, that actually women can be very well educated, that they can hold their own. Some of them have started small centres where women can study philosophy and have arranged for them to begin an academic program. Once it gets started, the momentum takes over, because these girls are intelligent, they are very devoted and they are very capable of learning. Once people begin to see that, they begin to take an interest and realize that there's this whole half of the population which up to now has been ignored. So even in the last ten years it's amazing. I mean previously you hardly saw any nuns anywhere; they were a non-presence. Now you see them all over, looking very bright, very confident, very capable. They are lovely girls.

LMN   So why in the past would a girl have become a nun?

TP   In Asia, you have two options: either you get married or you become a nun. For some girls, they just didn't want the household life. Their feeling was as a nun. Even though there were many disadvantages, nonetheless they were comparatively more free, and they could lead a life of virtue and pray hard, and next lifetime come back in a male body and become a monk.

LMN   The idea that only those in the male body can be enlightened is being widely challenged these days with so many Buddhist women starting to be teachers. You have vowed to attain Liberation as a woman and are now building a nunnery to support other women in their spiritual life. What will the nuns be learning?

TP   One of our plans is to re-establish what is called the Togdema lineage, which is a lineage of yoginis. Our monastery is very special in having a lineage of yogis (Togdens) who follow the Milarepa tradition, and in Tibet there were also the female equivalents, which now we don't have anymore. I think they were wiped out during the Cultural Revolution. If we can re-establish that with nuns who already have had a basic philosophical education and then on top of that they are doing profound practices, then I see no reason at all why in the future they shouldn't become well-qualified teachers. At the moment in the Tibetan tradition there is a great dearth of female teachers. I can only think of two female lamas in the Tibetan tradition. And both of them are closely connected with high lamas: one is a sister, one is a daughter of a very high lama. Both are very extraordinary and wonderful, but I mean two, only. So we need a few more.

LMN   It seems a lot easier for a Western woman to make her way up to being a respected spiritual teacher than it is for Asian women.

TP   Western women don't have the same social pressures. And because the Tibetans or the Indians don't expect anything of us anyway because we're not part of their social patterning, it leaves us very free. But I think now it's the time for the Asians themselves to begin to change their attitudes. And they are. It is therefore important to give the opportunity to these girls to study and get a sense of their own self-worth, their own qualities. Not to become proud, obviously, but just to have the confidence that they are capable of learning and experiencing, and realizing they are capable of giving and helping others. At the moment they don't have this because they always look to the monks and the lamas.

LMN   In the biography Cave in the Snow *you say you are primarily a contemplative practitioner. Now the work you are doing is putting you right out into the world. How did this change in focus happen?*

TP   Well, it wasn't something which I consciously chose. When I moved to Italy I tried at various points to set up retreat facilities and go into retreat, and every time there were very big obstacles, mostly physical obstacles, but absolutely a door slammed and said, no, that's not what you're supposed to be doing. So I really wondered what I was supposed to be doing. I thought, my whole life is given to the Buddha-Dharma-Sangha, what do you want? Then when I returned to Asia after five years, the lamas in my monastery said, look, we really need a nunnery, we don't have one, and so you please start one. Immediately I thought, yes, that's what I have to do. My own personal lama had previously said, I would like you to start a nunnery. In fact, he said that several times about twenty years ago, and I had just said, oh yes, and ignored it. But this time when the lamas said, you should start a nunnery, I thought, yes, now is the time.

So I then got catapulted into these world tours and things like this, which was the very last thing I would have ever considered myself ever, ever doing. But it's really been good. Being in retreat develops certain qualities, but being out in the world develops other qualities you could never develop in a retreat. So although it's absolutely not what I would have planned for myself, it's very interesting to see how one gets carried along into doing all sorts of things that one simply never would plan. Like being here now, meeting with officials, dealing with Indian bureaucracy, fundraising and dealing with accounts – all these things which I had never even given one thought to before. But that's how you learn, is it not?

LMN   What is it that you learn when you're out in the world compared to what you can learn in a cave?

TP   Well, in the cave you're there, and as I have often said, it's in a way like peeling off layers of the onion, one's usual identifications. When one is all by oneself, then playing at various identifications is kind of boring, so you begin to ask, who am I when I am not playing all these parts for people? Whatever parts one happens to be playing – we play so many. It's a much more introspective time. It's also a time for completely concentrating on a very set practice and becoming a pressure cooker in which all the energies and all the steam is building up and not leaking out, so that things can get cooked quite quickly.

When one is in the world, one has to develop other skills. There is more to the spiritual path than just meditation and introspection. There are also the qualities of generosity, patience, loving-kindness, compassion and so on, which you need to have other people around to develop. It's easy to sit in a cave thinking, may all beings be well and happy, but it's a different thing if you're out in the marketplace meeting these beings, many of whom are quite difficult to deal with. So that's when you really develop those kinds of social muscles.

One develops all sorts of qualities in a social context that one cannot develop alone, just as one develops many qualities alone that one couldn't develop in a social context. It's like breathing in and breathing out. We need to balance the two. I have certainly become more forthcoming. I think when I was living in the cave it was a little difficult to develop just how to be with other people. And now constantly traveling around, you know, learning how to stay focused and aware even in the middle of the marketplace is very important.

LMN   What do people want to know from you, now that your story is published?

TP   A lot of the people write to say they enjoyed the book and thank you and so on. I get a surprising number of letters from people who had quite profound spiritual experiences in their childhood or their adolescence, which completely transformed their whole view of what life is about and who they are. But they were living in a social context where nobody understood what they were talking about and thought they were nuts. Even if they went to their pastors or teachers, nobody knew what they were talking about. So a number of them went into quite a heavy psychological crisis because of this, because they were sure they had glimpsed something that was more real, but there was no endorsement from the environment and the culture around them. It's surprising how many letters I get from people who have had these kinds of experiences and are now so grateful to realize that what they had understood intuitively wasn't crazy after all. In fact, they really knew inside themselves that what they had experienced was extremely valid.

Of course, then the next question is: What do we do with it? How can we find a teacher? How can we find a path? This is always very difficult. How to advise people on that, I don't know. I do what I can depending on the individual and where they are, but it's very difficult nowadays for people to find authentic teachers. Or to find an authentic path which would suit them.

LMN   In your own journey to find a teacher, you met him fairly quickly.

TP   Yes, that was very smooth running. Many people don't have such good fortune. Also, in those days, if you did find your teacher you could be with them. Whereas nowadays, even if you find a teacher, they're never home. All these teachers are jet-setting around everywhere; it's very difficult for people. If you're lucky, you see them for five minutes once a year or something. Very difficult nowadays to create that genuine guru-chela relationship because the teachers are so elusive, really. They're spread so thin nowadays. Any teacher, especially if they speak English, ends up with thousands of disciples running all over here and there and everywhere and it's impossible to have a person-to-person relationship. This is a big problem. Whereas when I started, if you arrived in India and actually were interested in the dharma, all the doors were opened. They were so excited that a Westerner would be interested. Things have changed. So even though they didn't speak English, and they didn't really know what to teach you because they'd never had a Westerner before, nonetheless the contact was there. It was very easy to contact everybody, from the Dalai Lama downwards.

LMN How can teachers deal with this now? How is it going to have to change, with so many more disciples per teacher?

TP It's a problem. I think that what needs to be done is that, perhaps except in exceptional cases, people have to rely more on themselves and their own inner wisdom. Get the teachings, get the instructions, understand what they're supposed to be doing and then just settle down and do it, and make their own decisions. Person-to-person contact with teachers these days is very rare. I'm here at the moment in Dharamsala, which is a big Tibetan centre, and again and again I have long-term Western students coming and asking exactly this: How can I find a teacher? And here we are with hundreds and hundreds of monks and lamas, but to actually find a teacher and develop a relationship is not easy, even here.

LMN Do you see women in Buddhism taking more of a leadership role in the future? Would the nuns you are training perhaps become spiritual teachers?

TP Finally there is a recognition of this female element, and I think in the next ten years it will be very interesting to see what happens once these nuns who are just now studying graduate and become more mature figures, and to see what kind of voice they are going to have in the society. I think that will be very interesting. So to be a part of that is good, even though sometimes it seems an impossible task. But actually things are worthwhile. Because if we don't do it, nobody else is going to. The lamas are not going to do it. The women have to help each other, there's no doubt. To be part of that whole movement is nice. It's very strong at this time; the impetus is really flowing in full flood for helping these women. ॐ

[UPDATE: The Dongyu Gatsal Ling Nunnery is now established on three hectares of land overlooked by the majestic Dhauladhar mountain range. By the end of 2005 we will have over forty nuns from Tibet and other Himalayan regions who are studying Buddhist philosophy and practising meditation. Contrary to fears expressed in the interview, we have excellent monk teachers who are happy to be able to help with the nuns' education. The construction work for the nunnery is still in process, but the nuns are already living in the finished buildings on the land. We plan to eventually house 100 nuns. –Tenzin Palmo]

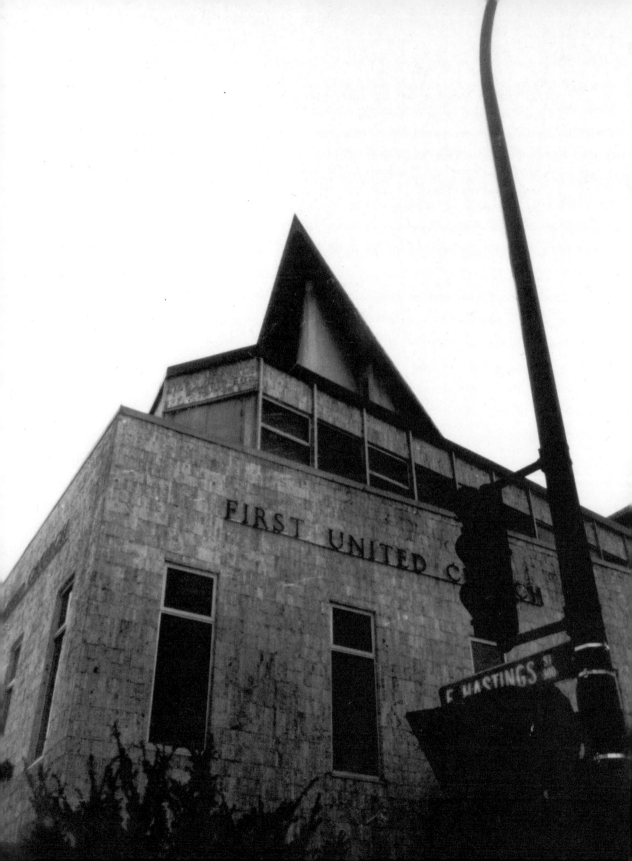

First published in Issue 5, Karma Yoga, Spring 2000

a day in the life of reverend ruth wright
ministering to the downtown eastside of vancouver

[by Reverend Ruth Wright]

Closing my apartment door, I hear my alarm clock ring. I fumble in my jacket pocket for the keys that will allow me to stop its noise before the neighbour's dog begins to howl. What is it about the clock that moves the dog to such a state? He didn't bark when I left the apartment an hour ago for my morning walk or when I came back either, but that 5:00 a.m. buzzer initiates an enraged response. All my good resolve to turn the alarm off when I first awaken gets lost in the trek to the shower, the donning of walking clothes, and the stillness of my meditation time.

The jolt of reality generated by the clock is a precursor of the stark reality of the early morning streets of Vancouver's downtown eastside (DTES). In contrast to the sleepy neighbourhoods of suburbia in the early morning hours, the streets in Canada's poorest urban community are abuzz with activity. Sex-trade workers wait on their corners for johns who worked late-night shifts. Pimps make their circuits, collecting the majority of the night's profits. Young children squat in

photo by Todd Stewart

alleys waiting for customers who will buy the drugs they flog. Men and women sleep in doorways, on steps of public buildings and in the parks – some are drunk, but more are homeless, mentally ill or physically challenged. My mind sometimes plays tricks on me and I think I am back in some parts of the developing world, surely not in Canada!

Driving into the parking lot of the First United Church, I count four people huddled on the steps to the entrance of the building. Their cardboard covers make it hard to know for sure, but I think there are three women and a man. As I walk toward them, I know I was right and I recognize two of their faces. Three are sleeping soundly, but the fourth is weeping quietly as she rubs her arm, which has obviously been injured. She is shivering violently from the dampness of the night on her worn cotton clothing. Sometimes I think Vancouver's wetness is harder to bear than the snowy cold of the north and east. A sugar-laced milky coffee and a wool blanket work their magic in minutes and I see her nodding off to sleep. The image of the "they" is gone and I see the unique face of a woman created by God. I hope when she awakens I can find her and learn her name – even if it's her street name. With a name, we can help her get the medical attention she needs and perhaps even help her find shelter for tonight.

It's 6:00 a.m. and the church is already busy. The smell of homemade soup stock and fresh-cut vegetables fills the building as they cook into a thick wholesome meal. The bread this morning is several days old, but it will be welcomed, broken and dunked in the broth by the 200 to 300 people who arrive for soup today. The thought of soup for breakfast day after day makes me shudder, but the folk in the soup line don't complain and even manage to joke: "Make mine oyster stew this morning!"

I watch with wonder at the patience of the people in our food line. They face another line for coffee, another for lunch and another for dinner. They may find themselves in a line waiting for clothing, for assistance from our paralegal advocates, for their mail, to use the telephone, to talk with a pastor, to get a blanket to cover themselves as they sleep in our pews, to get toiletries. Once again I am struck by the richness of choice that is mine and the limited choices people in poverty have.

There's poverty, and then there's poverty – even in this community. The chasm between the low-income residents with safe housing or single-room-occupancy hotels and those on the streets is as wide as the chasm between the rich and the poor. There is a distinct hierarchy even among the most destitute – prejudice is not the sole purview of the rich.

It's in the morning that I am most aware that the working backbone of this place is the DTES volunteers who come to make and serve soup, to stock the clothing room, to supervise the showers, and to do a variety of other tasks that need to be done in order for our programs to operate. They are wonderful people. Most of them have needed our help in the past, some need it now, but they are determined to make a contribution to this community through their volunteer work. The DTES volunteers work hand-in-hand with our other volunteers who come from all around the Greater Vancouver area. Some come daily, some once a week, others at particular seasons of the church year. They work with the gifts of food, clothing and funds offered by hundreds of people with a heart for the poor in the DTES. Many donors are church people who believe that God created us to be in community, to be kin, to care for one another and to seek justice for all.

At 8:45 six of us sit in a semi-circle around a piano bench at the front of the sanctuary in the building. A single candle reminds us of the presence of God's spirit, in this place and in each other. We read a passage of scripture, sing a hymn and pray together. Our service lasts fifteen minutes – a retreat in the midst of people sleeping on the pews, eating from their soup mugs, or talking quietly to one another. We move out into the day with the commission to "walk with justice, walk with mercy, and with God's humble care."

By 9:15 a long line of people has formed around the gym waiting for the coffee time to start. It's a time to have coffee or tea together and to visit. I hope to see the woman from our steps at coffee but she isn't there. As I walk through the building I am greeted by several people who want to chat for a few minutes. We share information about what is happening in the community, victories and failures. I am pleased that finally people are calling me Ruth, not "Reverend Ruth" or "Dr. Ruth." My academic mantle seems at last to have been shed.

The time "on the floor" talking with people who come for help and for company is the highlight of my day. I've heard rumours this morning that one of our regulars died alone in an alley last night. Her street brothers and sisters will soon be looking for staff to talk with about their loss of yet another friend. I know that someone will come today to ask that we have a memorial service soon. We will certainly celebrate her life – but first the coroner's office will have to confirm the death and we will try to contact the family and learn where the body or ashes will be sent – then we are free to plan the service with the help of her best friends.

These services are wonderfully uplifting events. In the midst of all the sadness and loss, we hear again and again how the people on the streets help each other, become family, love and care for each other! When I hold a weeping friend in my arms, hear an elder speak with wisdom, experience the heartlike rhythm of a First Nations drummer, or feel the comforting repetitiveness of a singer, my faith in a Creator is strengthened. I hear the fear of being alone in death, and I know the importance of building community in this place.

The provincial government has reshuffled its cabinet and changed the name of the ministry which our advocates work with most often. We have come to distrust those changes because they have so frequently foreshadowed additional red tape through which the poor and the unhealthy have to find their way to survive. Each of these changes increases the pressure on our advocates, whose caseloads are already more than they can handle. Some agencies in the community have decided to take a public stand against the coming changes. The remainder of my morning is spent in meetings with their representatives.

After lunch, the morning's messages are still on my voicemail to be dealt with: a youth leader who wants to bring a group of young adults for an awareness day in the DTES; a community group wanting us to contribute money for a local art show; an instructor from a local college wanting us to provide a placement site for a student; a Rotary group offering to donate a burial plot to us; a minister inviting me to preach at another church, so parishioners there will understand why we ask for food and funds from them; a reporter wanting a reaction to the disappearance of another sex-trade worker; a donor wanting to know why we used environmentally unfriendly labels on a mailing a year ago; a woman wanting us to find her brother, who she thinks is living on the streets here; and a colleague wanting to "do lunch" to talk about strategies to encourage the development of more detox treatment beds for women in this area. My first thoughts are that there is no room in my calendar for any of this, but I know full well that there must and will be time.

I spend the afternoon preparing for an upcoming board meeting, checking with the financial officer about the state of our accounts, writing letters to potential donors, and checking in with a staff member whose health is a major concern for me right now. The staff member seems to be doing better than the budget, and there are some restless moments and rapid heartbeats as I review the figures and find that costs are escalating and our donations are not! I'm a teacher, an administrator, an academic and a minister by training, not a fundraiser – yet somehow it is a major part of my job. But that's another front on which faith plays an important role – there has been a church presence on this corner for 115 years. Our vision of outreach has been part of the ethos of the community since the Depression, and if we are meant to continue this work in this place, a way will be found.

It is ironic that our very reason for being in a community like this is to work ourselves out of a job, and though we are working harder and harder we are needed more, not less. How can it be that after all those years have passed, the poor are worse off than they ever were, there are more and more people finding it impossible to survive without help, and our social policies are making facilities like ours more and more necessary for people's survival?

Our mission statement is simple. It says we are called by the Spirit to be a part of the DTES of Vancouver to affirm the growth of the individual, to enable community and to work for social justice. Community grows when people respect each other, when they are known by name, when their input and opinions are valued, no matter how diverse. From community comes the voice that is strong enough to evoke social justice. As I look around the community I see lots of evidence that this place has played a significant role in the community. It has been the birthplace for the Downtown Eastside Residents Association, the First United Church Social Housing Society, the Downtown Eastside Handicapped Association, and a major player in the birth of Crab Tree Corner, the Lookout and a handful of other agencies working successfully in this community, strengthening it.

A telephone call just as I am leaving is as jolting as the alarm clock this morning. It is from a merchant who is angry at people sleeping in his doorway, urinating in the alleyway near his shop, and using the area as a drug-shooting gallery. His anger that the poor, the homeless, the addicted and the abused are allowed to come to our building – to his neighbourhood – is real and to some extent understandable. While I listen to his angry criticism of our presence in this community, it is difficult not to retaliate with comments about the under-the-counter sale of rice wine in shops like his, which has killed so many people in this community. His anger begins to dissipate as we talk about the need for drug and alcohol treatment centres, but he is very clear that they should be somewhere other than this neighbourhood.

I know this man is a generous person and that he helps a lot of people in his own quiet way. I can understand his frustration with the large numbers of people who hang out in places like First. On his good days he understands the need for the work we do, but at other times the negatives of our presence are foremost in his mind. He doesn't agree with our practice of allowing people who are intoxicated or high to sleep in our pews, yet he is appalled by the numbers of deaths in alleys. He thinks we go too far in our open-door policies.

As I talk with him I have images of dead people – people who have overdosed and died on our steps – who have been brought back to life by injections of Narcan. I see emergency response teams working frantically to bring back dozens of people and I am sure that it is our call to allow as few people to die as possible. I can talk of hard-nosed practices, in principle, but I cannot look into the face of any person and say in my heart that they deserve to die because they are an alcoholic, a drug addict, mentally ill or poor.

My watch reads 6:30 p.m. as I leave the building for a meeting in the west end of the city. It's a meeting of ministers and representatives from United churches in our Presbytery. I've missed the meal we eat together seven times each year, but there will be opportunity to speak about the work at the First United later in the evening. With good chairing, we should be on our way home by 9:00 p.m. I look forward to some time to walk, to read scripture and to journal before setting the alarm for tomorrow's start. ॐ

The human spirit needs to be fed as much as the human body needs to be fed. So my hope is the tide will turn and darkness will be extinguished by lighting many many candles around the world. That is my hope.

First published in Issue 9, The Environment, Spring 2001

it takes a genius to be simple
a profile of satish kumar

[by Lesley Marian Neilson]

Outside the window a light snow is falling. It catches on the cedar and pine trees and settles on the hard ground. I have just put a call through to England, to the home of Satish Kumar. He and his wife June edit *Resurgence,* a magazine of spiritual and ecological thought, out of the same kitchen in which they eat, entertain, drink a cup of tea. Satish's voice comes crackly over the phone line. As we talk, I watch the snowfall and at the same time try to picture what might be outside his window. Occasionally I hear other voices in the background, the people he works with to put out the magazine. He has just returned from spending December in India and no doubt there is a lot of work to catch up on.

I first came across Satish Kumar in a profile written by Jay Walljasper, published in *Utne Reader.* Walljasper is a contributor to *Resurgence,* and in the profile he is in part searching for the reason he agrees to write a column for *Resurgence* for no pay. He explains that "to say no to Satish, who speaks in an elegant, melodious flow of Indian-accented English, would feel like turning down a prestigious, hard-won honour. No one published in *Resurgence* has ever seen a pence for their labours, and the list includes luminaries like Václav Havel, Gary Snyder, Ted Hughes, James Hillman, Winona LaDuke, Wendell Berry, Susan Griffin, Ivan Illich, and Noam Chomsky."

I was struck by the description of how Satish integrates work, relaxation, community, beauty and appreciation of nature into a self-described "simple" lifestyle. Nothing is more inspiring than people who live actively by their ideals, who strive for and attain balance and peace. Painting a picture of Satish's home, Walljasper writes:

"By almost any economic standard of the modern world they are poor, yet it's almost impossible not to envy their life. Meals usually come straight from the garden. The centuries-old cottage lacks central heat but is as comfortable as any home I've set foot in; it's outfitted with furnishings, kitchenware, and art that embody the rustic elegance that *Martha Stewart Living* magazine and the Pottery Barn strive for. The long table in the middle of the wood-beamed kitchen, where friends and family gather over Satish's Indian dinners and June's desserts, drinking local cider and talking for hours, feels like the centre of the universe."

When I was a kid and imagined my life as an adult, I dreamt of living on a farm, surrounded by nature and animals, and having a classical mansion for my house. It seemed the perfect compromise between my love of the natural world and my desire for material comfort. As I've grown older, the dream has remained remarkably constant, with only one significant change: the mansion has been razed and replaced with a more modest dwelling, ideally one that I have built myself.

I call this dream a pursuit of self-sufficiency – an idea that is constantly being formed and reformed by my understanding of what sustains me, my family, my community, the planet. It's an idea that Satish has spent his life exploring, and about which he has much to say.

"Self-sufficiency begins with self-satisfaction and contentment within, rather than looking for contentment from outside stimulation and gratification. So self-sufficiency is, first of all, to be contented within oneself.

"The second part [of self-sufficiency] is to be satisfied with what you have already. We are always looking for something new, something different, something more, and do not value what is already there.

"The third part of self-sufficiency is to be able to use one's own skills and one's own resources to make things – being able to cook your own food, rather than always depending on somebody else to cook for you or going out to restaurants. The basic skills of living are very important.

"When we are talking about food, it's not only cooking, but also a little bit of growing, a little garden where food, vegetables and herbs and that sort of thing can be grown. Then you are appreciating what is around you, you have a sense of place and have some connection with the natural world. That way you are using and developing your own skills, your own hands, and you are also not being dependent on your entertainment, your knowledge, your ideas on faraway things, but appreciating what is local. So local is important for a simple self-sufficient life.

"And then [self-sufficiency means] finding ways of living that have means of good health – for example, yoga and meditation and going for a walk in your area. If your health is good, you are not dependent on medicine and hospitals and doctors and other sorts of treatments. So these are the basic elements of self-sufficiency that support and enhance and nourish your simple life."

Many people I have talked to have the idea that self-sufficiency requires being completely independent from everyone else, perhaps living in a cabin in a forest, gathering roots and berries and hunting animals. This vision is not only extreme, it misses one of the basics points of self-sufficiency: to live in sustainable harmony with the Earth, the community and oneself. Strong human relationships and physical work are the basis of self-sufficiency.

"First of all," says Satish, "you need to develop a relationship with your own being. Sometimes we don't appreciate ourselves, and we don't know who we are, so we are dissatisfied within ourselves and are always looking for outside [approval]. Once you are able to relate to yourself, then you start relating through your skills with your surrounding. You relate with your land, you relate with trees, you relate with flowers, you relate with the stream at the bottom of your garden, you relate to the natural world. And then you are able to relate to your community. No human being is an island by himself or herself. We exist in a web of relationships, not in isolation.

"The idea of Descartes was that *I think, therefore I am,* which means I am just an isolated individual and not connected. Whereas my thinking is that self-

sufficiency exists within community, within relationship. It's not I think, therefore
I am, but you are, therefore I am; trees are, therefore I am; the community is,
therefore I am. Simplicity and self-sufficiency are embedded in relationship."

Satish is one of the foremost advocates of the ideas of E.F. Schumacher, the
ecological economist most widely known for his 1973 book, *Small Is Beautiful.*
Schumacher's ideas hinge on the principles of appropriate technologies and
human-scale economies. In his lifetime, Schumacher wrote numerous articles for
Resurgence, practised his ideas through small-scale living, by which he grew his
own food and used technology only as a way to enhance his own work, rather than
to make his labour obsolete. His example was pivotal in focusing Satish's lifelong
activism on the furthering of ecological and spiritual values through education
and lifestyle choice. Their meeting was, as Satish writes in his autobiography
Path Without Destination, "instantly a meeting of minds, and the beginning of a
friendship that was to last beyond his death."

Satish first met Schumacher in 1968, shortly after the economist published
an essay entitled "Buddhist Economics." Schumacher had put these two seemingly
disparate systems of thought together while in Burma on assignment for the
British government. Not only did he see that the Burmese had an economic
system that harmonized their cultural beliefs with their material needs, but
that traditional economics could in fact learn significant lessons from Buddhist
principles. "The Buddhist point of view," Schumacher writes, "takes the function
of work to be at least threefold: to give a man a chance to utilize and develop his
faculties; to enable him to overcome his ego-centredness by joining with other
people in a common task; and to bring forth the goods and services needed for a
becoming existence."

Throughout *Small Is Beautiful,* Schumacher links the increasing social
atmosphere of depression, disempowerment and disability to the decrease in
imaginative and physical work. "The type of work that modern technology is
most successful in reducing or even eliminating," he writes, "is skillful, productive
work of human hands, in touch with real materials of one kind or another. In an
advanced industrial society, such work has become exceedingly rare, and to make a
decent living by doing such work has become virtually impossible. A great part of
the modern neurosis may be due to this very fact; for the human being, defined by

Thomas Aquinas as a being with brains and hands, enjoys nothing more than to be creatively, usefully, productively engaged with both his hands and his brains."

These words resonate with particular power for me. Recently I quit my job and moved away from Toronto, where I have worked for a year in offices, doing nothing much at all. On the rare occasions I was given the chance to use my mind and creativity I jumped at it, but those moments could not counteract the increasing resentment I felt and the growing sense that my intelligence was draining away. When Satish says over the phone, "If you don't work, then your imagination is not nurtured; and when you don't do anything, then your imagination goes dry, gets hungry and goes under," I know exactly what he is talking about. There were times when I felt as if I was drowning.

"The thing about self-sufficiency and simplicity," says Satish, "is that both these ideas are only possible when we begin to appreciate the sacred quality and fulfilling quality of work. A human body is naturally in need of work, so if we stop doing productive work, creative work, then we begin to do unnecessary and unproductive and uncreative work. So working on the garden and making things by hand and seeing it as sacred work is vital – not as work just to earn money or just to keep your body and soul together, but work that is an expression of beauty, an expression of service, an expression of gift.

"When you are a craftsperson and take a lump of clay, you discover that that lump of clay has a pot in it. Or you take a piece of wood and uncover a beautiful chair in it. Or you take a lump of stone and you uncover a beautiful image, a statue in it. So only through work you can uncover and discover and unfold the beauty and the sacred. You make something which is beautiful, which is useful, which is dutiful, which is a gift and which is something that can last."

"But how do we start to uncover the sacred," I ask, "if we are already caught up in the material, modern, technological world?"

"You begin small. If you are living in the city, then you begin with having a few plants in your window, on your balcony and on your rooftop. That way you are connecting with the natural world. Then you begin to use what you have grown – a few herbs, a few vegetables – and you cook them. And when you are cooking you are starting to work. Then you say, can I, even in the city, can I do some tapestry, can I do some weaving, can I do some knitting? Can I do something that expresses my deep core of feelings and imagination?"

Beauty is a quality neither Schumacher nor Satish underestimates. Bring art, poetry and imagination into your home, Satish says. It is inhuman to simply go to work, spend long hours commuting, and then sit in front of the television. "That is not the idea of simple life, which has self-sufficiency and creativity and sacred enshrined in it."

Satish has spent his whole life as an activist, learning what is worth fighting for, and how to merge his spiritual and political beliefs. Born in India in 1936, he grew up in an intensely spiritual culture in the midst of a century of unprecedented change. He has witnessed the world spin steadily faster, become smaller through improved communications and also become more and more threatened by the life choices of the affluent societies. Since he was a small boy his feet have been in intimate contact with the earth, and so, rooted by his spiritual beliefs, he fights for the preservation of the planet on which his feet walk.

As a nine-year-old boy in his native India, Satish took vows of renunciation and became a Jain monk. For eight years he wandered through India with a begging bowl and little else, until he was introduced to Gandhi's philosophy. "What Gandhi was saying," Satish writes, "was that religion is not religion if it does not help to solve the problems of this world, here and now." Leaving his Jain brotherhood, Satish spent two years walking with Vinoba, Gandhi's foremost disciple, convincing landowners to donate land to the landless.

By now Satish's feet were hard, his legs strong; he had spent most of his life walking. And he was learning about political action.

A few years after leaving Vinoba, Satish set off on his most ambitious walk ever. It was 1962 and antinuclear demonstrations were heating up around the world. In England, Bertrand Russell had been arrested for protesting, inspiring Satish to think once again of nonviolent political action. He had read the news of Russell's protest in an English paper, brought to him by his friend Prabhakar Menon, and over coffee the two decided on an action of their own: to walk from India to Washington on a Peace Pilgrimage. They would visit the nuclear capitals and impress upon Khrushchev, de Gaulle, Wilson and Johnson a message of peace. On June 1, they stood at Gandhi's gravesite and began their journey. Over the next eighteen months, the two friends walked through India, Pakistan, Afghanistan, Iran, the Soviet Union, northern Europe to England, crossed the Atlantic by boat and ended their pilgrimage at John F. Kennedy's grave in Washington.

Over the next seven years, Satish walked in Italy and in India again. He wrote and edited magazines and lived in the forest. He consulted a *sadhu* who said, "Very soon you are going on a long journey over the ocean....Once you are in the far land, you are going to meet someone in that land who will completely change your life."

Having just returned from Europe, Satish was certain he was not heading off on another journey, but soon after the *sadhu*'s predictions, he was invited to England to put on an exhibition about the war in Bangladesh and the mass exodus of refugees into India. While putting on the exhibit, Satish met June. After touring Europe he returned to England to find her, and they are together still, with their two children. England became Satish's adopted home and there he was able to settle in a way never before possible for him.

Satish and June have been editing *Resurgence* for twenty-five years. At first they lived in London, with a small garden, but eventually decided to move away from the moneyed lifestyle of the city. By this point, they were already dedicated to the ideals of community, self-sufficiency and local economies. After an initial experiment in communal living fell apart, Satish, June and their two children, Mukti and Maya, moved onto a few acres of property in Hartland in rural north Devon.

"We planted a couple of hundred trees of all kinds. Some trees for wood, some trees for herbs, some trees for fruit, some trees for furniture – all kinds of trees, like ash and oak and willows and apple and pear and so on. Also we have a garden, so we can live and work and garden from our home."

From there, Satish became involved in a successful experiment in education, starting a Small School in Hartland, a community which he describes in *Path Without Destination* as being "almost self-sufficient as a village." Until the Small School, the only option for children over the age of eleven was to commute long distances to go to school in larger towns. Not only were the classrooms in the larger schools crowded and impersonal, the arrangement "also gave the children the idea that the village was not good enough for them, as it could not provide the necessary education, and when they finished their education it would not provide them with work."

The school that Satish and a group of interested parents started combined the traditional academic subjects with creative and practical skills. The children help build, cook and garden, and emerge from their education with both intellectual and physical skills that can carry them solidly into their adult life.

In the late 1980s Satish became involved in another project in education, this time the development of a college of holistic science. Schumacher College opened in 1991, and is dedicated to teaching and advancing the ideas of spiritual ecology that have been explored in the pages of *Resurgence* for decades. Satish became the director of the college, while continuing to edit the magazine. In his autobiography he writes: "Schumacher College is the culmination of my life's work. Here it is possible to bring together the spiritual foundation of the monk's life, the social concerns of the Bhoodan movement, the ideals of peace that I pursued during my walk around the world, and the ecological concerns of *Resurgence*. This is a convergence of the values and aspirations by which I have been guided throughout my life."

Looking back, I can mark my path by the revolutionary ideas that made me rise a little in consciousness. Through the down-to-earth, practical application of his spiritual and ecological beliefs, Satish Kumar represents a revolution in my own thinking and living. "What," I ask him, "have been the most influential ideas you have encountered in the past thirty years?"

"Small is beautiful is the first idea that I encountered, and E.F. Schumacher started that. It is still not yet quite popular enough, although the book has been read and 'small is beautiful' has become part of our language, but still people are hell-bent on growing growing growing. Big hospitals, big schools, big government, big buildings, high-rise, big companies, multinationals, transnationals, globalization – all that is a trend toward bigness. Whereas the most pertinent and most exciting and revolutionary idea is small is beautiful.

"Then the idea that Gregory Bateson and various other people developed that everything is a system. We are all part of systems. We are all connected. Systems thinking to me was a very important idea in which everything is connected, everything is mutually dependent on each other. When you look at something, you have to see it in relationship with everything else. We are dependent on the earth; we are dependent on the air, water, fire.

"And from systems thinking emerges the Gaia Theory, which is James Lovelock's idea, in which the whole Earth is one living organism and we are part of the web of life and human beings are not superior.

"That leads to deep ecology – accepting the intrinsic value of all life. The trees have intrinsic value. Animals have intrinsic value. The forests have intrinsic value. The Earth as a living system comes from Gaia, and then the intrinsic value of all life comes from deep ecology.

"And that leads of course to the idea of permaculture. How every way we live, our energy system, our food system, our work system should all be such that it's dutiful, permanent and sustainable. So from systems thinking to Gaia to deep ecology to permaculture to sustainability – these are some of the seminal ideas that have inspired me and *Resurgence*."

When I lived in Toronto, I had to take a step back from my convictions as an environmentalist; otherwise, it was too frustrating living in a city where pollution hangs so thickly in the air I can taste it, where cars are noisy, indispensable ornaments that make biking a health hazard, where each day the garbage piles up on the curb and city council thinks it's a good idea to ship the garbage to a defunct mine in a small northern community. As a city dweller, I depended on the outlying agricultural areas to provide my food, faraway hydroelectric projects to provide my energy, and a vast governmental infrastructure to maintain my roads, water, social services and economy. Giant billboard ads for the downtown shopping centre read: People say Torontonians think they are the centre of the universe. They are!

"I think," says Satish, "that there is at the moment in the world a battle going on between those who are pursuing materialistic paths – globalizers of economic growth and those hell-bent on this 'big is better' idea – on the one hand, and on the other hand those who are dedicated to spiritual renewal, more small-scale development, more human scale, more sustainability, more crafts and arts. Where human beings are not just sold to companies and money and those kinds of things. Where human beings have a sacred path.

"These two forces are in a way like the battlefield in the Bhagavad Gita, where Arjuna and Krishna were fighting the Kauravas. This battlefield is still with us, it's in every generation, in every situation that is going on, but at this moment it is the materialism on the one hand and the spiritual values and more ecological lifestyle on the other. At the moment, media, money, advertising and governments are all behind the materialistic globalization, but the people are not feeling very happy.

"There's a kind of a depression going on, and people are unhealthy, and people are realizing it's stressful, this treadmill, this strenuous lifestyle, and we are being forced to earn earn earn and not live and enjoy and celebrate life. So people are standing up like in the Seattle and Washington protests against the World Bank and IMF [International Monetary Fund] and WTO [World Trade Organisation], and the Prague demonstration and protest, and the protest against the world debt system. This battle is almost a worldwide civil war and in the next ten years I think the forces of more spiritual and ecological and sustainable and small scale and simple and self-sufficient lifestyle should get a bit stronger. That I can say with more hope than I can predict anything; I don't know what is going to happen. But I am dedicating my life to support that alternative."

The snow is still falling outside the window, but I am smiling at the speakerphone, out of which Satish's voice rises. His words are energizing, gentle, wise. He is not an angry man, despite the Goliath forces we are up against.

"What do you hope for?" I ask.

"I hope that the human spirit will rise. I hope that human beings are not going to allow themselves to be swallowed by the forces of economic growth and the materialistic paradigm, because the human life is much more than high-rise buildings and motorcars and highways and airports and cyberspace. Human life needs relationships, love, compassion, caring friendships, generosity, time to read, time to study, time to meditate, time to go for walks, explore mountains and forests and rivers – to be rather than have and do. The human spirit needs to be fed as much as the human body needs to be fed. So my hope is the tide will turn and darkness will be extinguished by lighting many many candles around the world. That is my hope." ॐ

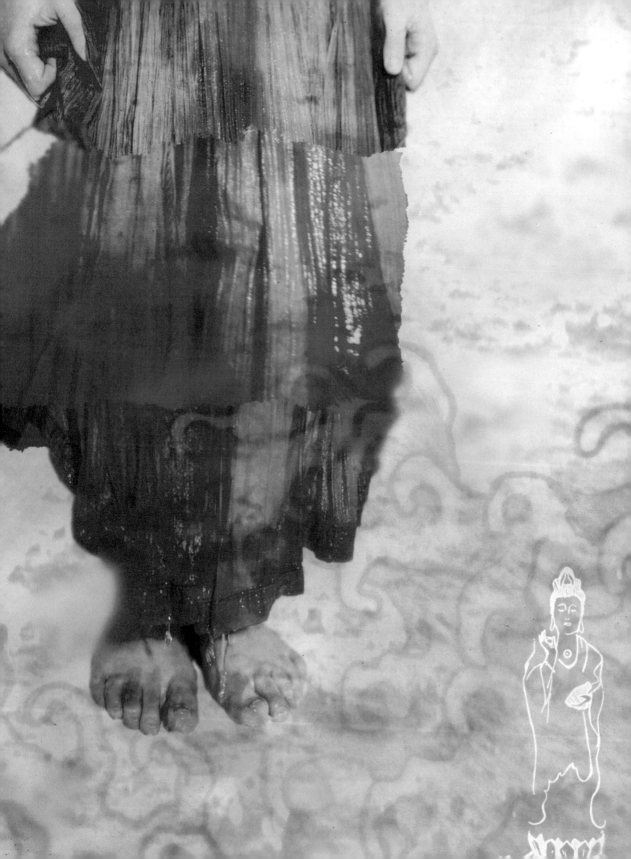

First published in Issue 13, Life & Death, Spring 2002

the blessed & cursed catastrophe we call death & dying
a practice of engagement

[Joan Halifax Roshi interviewed by Clea McDougall]

It is a quiet and early morning. I shut the door to my yellow room. After nearly a month of trying to arrange a time that would fit into our busy schedules, the call to Joan Halifax goes through easily this morning. She answers right away. Finally, from sunlit and snowy Montréal, I reach what must be a place of ochres and browns and sands: Santa Fe.

Joan Halifax Roshi is inspiring what she calls a gentle revolution in dying. A Buddhist teacher, author, anthropologist and social activist, she is the founder of the Upaya Zen Centre, a Buddhist study centre committed to teaching and practising the contemplative care of the dying. The centre reaches out into the community with projects such as Being with Dying, which teaches health professionals, caregivers and people with severe illnesses contemplative perspectives on death and dying, as well as offering retreats that emphasize "the awareness of death as the ground for the experience of dying and of caring for life." Their Partners Program trains volunteers to sit with the dying, and the Upaya Prison

illustration by Emrys Damon Miller

Project brings this work to prisoners on death row.

Joan is also one of the main proponents of engaged spirituality, a movement that supports new ways of practising compassionate action in the world.

Through all the action in her life, Joan still manages to speak from a place of stillness. As we talk there are the long full silences of a woman who has trained her mind through sitting with herself and with the dying. I listen closely this morning to her words and her silent spaces.

Joan Halifax Roshi's life has a remarkable balance of ordinariness and extraordinariness. When I ask her what a day of her life at Upaya is like, she responds, "I sit in the *zendo,* I teach, I sit with dying people, I garden, I write, I clean. It's a regular life. I'm very fortunate to live in an extremely beautiful place, but we are surrounded by suffering, so I have to ask, how can I bring the gifts of my life forward to really help other beings?"

"And how do you do this?" I ask.

"I sit with people literally all over the world, around this particular blessed and cursed catastrophe we call death and dying."

Clea McDougall   What drew you to work with the dying?

Joan Halifax Roshi   I think it was my grandmother who gave me a heart for working with dying people. She was from Savanna, Georgia and was a sculptress. Many of the beautiful monuments in the Bonaventure cemetery in Savanna were made by her. She had a great deal of peace with dying and transmitted to me the depth of experience in being present for a dying person.

CM   And what made you follow it through into your spiritual life?

JHR   I think that my interest in being with the dying comes out of my own suffering. I am reminded that suffering is part of the experience of profound transformation that one goes through on a spiritual journey. You can learn a lot from people and from yourself when you observe the inevitability of death, your own responses and the responses of others to that truth, that fact.

CM   What can we learn about life through observing death?

JHR In Zen, we call the great question Life *and* Death. There's no real separation between the two. To be fully in life is to also be fully in death. At a point, the mind stops making personality statements; there is cessation in terms of what we do, who we think we are, what we think the world is. When you're with a dying person, your own priorities change dramatically. Death is a very profound experience to be close to. It is the experience of that which is really ungraspable and ultimately uncontrollable.

CM You've referred to the people you work with, the dying, as bodhisattvas. *Why?*

JHR Because they really teach one compassion.

CM Yet your work gives so much to the dying… it seems like a process of give and take. Would you consider yourself a bodhisattva?

JHR Oh, not at all. I'm an aspiring one. But I'm also very much a human being with many flaws and many challenges. And the work feels beyond give and take. It's more a quality of open presence to whatever is arising.

CM You have used the image of the bodhisattva *riding the waves of birth and death when talking about impermanence. Why is it so hard for people to accept change, or accept the idea of impermanence?*

JHR It's an inability to accept the groundlessness of existence – the fact that you can't hold onto anything. We tend to fixate on a lover or a religion or an idea or a place, and that fixation is a source of suffering. When you come to the situation realizing that nothing stays, then you have a certain kind of freedom.

CM Is that freedom ever really attainable? Just when I start to think I understand impermanence, something comes up that makes me realize that I haven't accepted it fully. Do you think we can ever get to that point of freedom? Are you at that point?

JHR I think there are moments when I am there and moments when I am not there. The whole practice is about opening yourself to a basic not knowing, to being with the inconceivable and not trying to figure it all out. And that is, in essence, what the practice of being with the dying is all about for me. You don't know; you bear witness to each moment as it arises. The image of riding the waves of birth and death shows that you are in a continuum of constant change, constant groundlessness. And instead of drowning in the waters you are surfing, you are riding it. And every time you fixate, you start to drown. The struggle can be very profound. And that includes when we are dying and grasping onto life.

CM *You've quoted Rilke: "Love and death are the greatest gifts given to us, but mostly they are passed on unopened." So what would we find if we opened the gift of love and the gift of death?*

JHR Each person finds what is theirs, and it changes through time, as well. The fact is that love and death are about fully letting go. Rilke brings it to a beautiful characterization when he talks about these great gifts that are given to us. In the Middle Ages, the Christian monks bent over and whispered in each other's ears – *memento mori* – remember death. Spiritual practitioners the world over have used death as a way to deepen their lives. I think it's an extraordinary opportunity for each of us to observe those who are dying in order to not just help them, but to liberate ourselves from the continuum of suffering.

CM *Can you talk a bit about engaged spirituality?*

JHR Engaged spirituality, in the best sense, means that we simply are in the world helping other beings seamlessly. It's not just sort of frantically helping another being, it is a contemplative practice. We can use our service to others and say this situation is actually my practice. And I think that can be really great. There can be a big problem in engaged spirituality if there is an intent to do good in the world. You have to be very careful that it's not some kind of socially prescribed or socially winning behaviour.

From the Mahayana perspective, engagement means you are constantly looking with experience and compassion as a basis for your practice. And compassion is different from sympathy or pity. It's really being able to feel the suffering of others and also to see the source of their suffering, which is usually a delusion, and to try to help people transform delusion into something else.

CM *And how would people be able to start making their practices engaged?*

JHR Well, I think there are many ways to do it. To begin with, you need to have some kind of contemplative practice that allows the mind to become stable and that cultivates compassion and then insight. And once you have those elements present, when you can do your work with stability, then you translate your practice into the world. And that's really the point. In Zen we say, "Before enlightenment, chop wood and carry water. After enlightenment, chop wood and carry water." It's the same activity, but it's done in a very different way. The emphasis is on service as a spiritual path but not a path of ego.

CM *What is the path of service?*

JHR I think it is the realization that all beings are interconnected at the most fundamental level. So, if you are "serving" another person you are really serving yourself, and the more your ego gets out of the way the better you can do it. It's a great experience to be in a relaxed, seamless relationship with the world and it's not "service" – you've gotten over the syndrome of the server, where A is doing something for B. Some Buddhists use the image of the right hand taking care of the left hand, because it happens automatically. It's a question of whether you can open yourself to that degree.

CM *You've brought your work into prisons. What has that been like?*

JHR It's been an extraordinarily deep experience, working with people in prison systems. We work a lot in death row and maximum security, where you become a companion to hopelessness. You can't hope for any outcome, because usually the outcomes are pretty similar – death or life incarceration. But without the typical expectations, you have greater freedom in the kind of work that you do.

CM *Can I ask what you do when you sit with people who are dying?*

JHR It really depends on the individual. There is no prescription except being present, to be fully present. There can't be a prescription because every individual and every moment is unique, so having a practice that really stabilizes

the blessed & cursed catastrophe we call death & dying 59

you is critical in this regard. You may have to rub a foot or a head, or change a bedpan or counsel the dying person or be with family members or facilitate good communication with the family or help educate the family around the issues, or help the family make decisions that are helpful… it's a constant process that is unpredictable. So you have to be present and at the ready and not afraid.

CM It must be a very intense way to engage in life, to be present with death constantly.

JHR Well, I think it's rather liberating. I'd rather be examining these deep questions and constantly waking up to reality in this way than to sleep my life away. ॐ

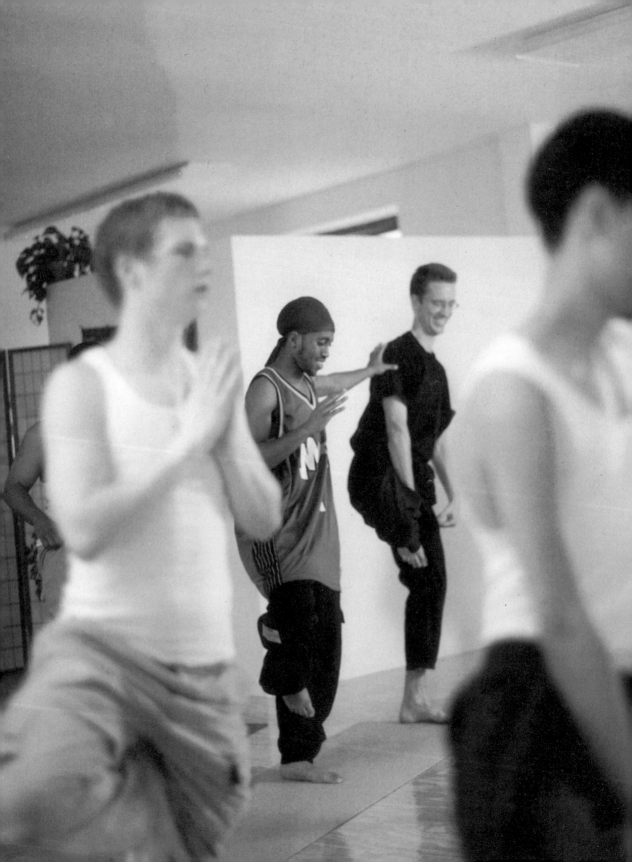

First published in Issue 10, Bhakti, Summer 2001

accident prone
bringing yoga to the bronx

[by Soren Gordhamer]

t his is bullshit," says Michael, a fifteen-year-old boy who is at my class for the first time. We have just finished twenty minutes of yoga and are now sitting down for meditation. I'm in the middle of one of the eight meditation and yoga classes I teach each week for incarcerated teens in New York City Juvenile Halls. These juvenile facilities are located in the poorest neighbourhoods of the Bronx, Brooklyn and Harlem. The youth are primarily fourteen- to sixteen-year olds from the inner city who have lived very dangerous lives: they have been shot at, chased by the cops and in numerous fights. At a very young age they have often both endured and caused great amounts of suffering. Some of them are members of the Bloods, Crips or similar gangs. Sometimes kids get involved because the gangs control the drug business in the inner city and this is how the youth make money. Other kids join for protection, saying it is unsafe not to have a gang affiliation.

I've been interested in working with teens ever since I went through the

photo courtesy the Lineage Project

passage myself some years ago. Depressed and lonely as a teenager, my father often left books outside my door that he thought I should read. These books were usually on sexuality or spiritual practice – maybe the two most difficult subjects for children and parents to discuss. Growing up as one of the few non-churchgoers in the Bible Belt of West Texas, my parents wanted to introduce my siblings and me to a number of different traditions. My mom was a yoga practitioner and later a yoga teacher. My father was a psychologist with an interest in meditation. I began meditation and yoga from a young age, though I mainly did the practices by myself in my room and tried to keep it from my parents. Heaven forbid they find out that I was taking some of their advice!

About ten years later, there came a point in my practice when I felt a strong desire to offer these practices to youth. If it helped me, I thought, surely it could help other young people. I had a few friends who were meditators and had been incarcerated as teenagers, so we decided to begin the experiment at the local juvenile hall where they were once incarcerated.

After several years working at facilities in the San Francisco Bay area, I moved to New York City a little over a year ago to begin programs for youth in one of America's toughest cities. The nonprofit group I direct is called the Lineage Project East. We offer classes that consist of meditations, such as mindfulness of breathing and listening to Tibetan bells; simple and easy yoga stretches that help them gently contact and move their bodies; teaching stories and dharma topics; along with a discussion period. Everything the Lineage Project offers in the classes is in the spirit of supporting more awareness or mindfulness, encouraging in the youth a sense of curiosity and exploration.

Classes over the last year have become easier as more and more kids have become accustomed to our programs. The kids who end up in juvenile hall come in with enormous confusion and emotional pain. They desperately want help but are extremely suspicious of everybody. Whenever I start a new class, there is usually a "feel out" stage. This involves the kids insulting both the practices and me, then watching how I respond. "You ever been told you look like that guy from *Ghostbusters*, Egon. Nah, you look like Slinky man. This meditation stuff is dumb. People really like to do this? I can't believe how stupid this stuff is." Sometimes these comments express legitimate doubt about the class, but mainly they are putting me through an initiation. Can I be insulted? How do I respond when the practices I hold dear are criticized? Their central question seems to be,

"Do I care about them more than I care about them doing meditation and yoga?"

With Michael, the kid who thinks this is bullshit, I tell him that I'm not here to fix or lecture him, but that I will explore with him ways to improve the situation he is in. "We will be doing some practices," I explain. "If they are not useful, then forget about them. Don't take my word for it. See for yourself if they have any benefit. But if you never try something, you'll never know." He looks at me with a little more interest, but like most of the kids in this facility, he struggles with enormous pain – of friends killed in gang violence, parents in prison, extreme poverty, few vocational choices that offer any future, and a neighbourhood plagued by violence. They wonder if they start opening to this pain, where will it end? Is it even worth it?

All the so-called "troublemakers" in the city end up in one of three juvenile centres. The juvenile centres are large buildings that hold about 125 youth each, and are often the newest and most expensive buildings in the entire neighbourhood. Security at the facilities is very tight, and all visitors are searched and put through a metal detector. The kids all wear large beige jumpers and have to ask to do anything, even go to the bathroom. They walk in single-file lines through the halls, and must count off as they enter and leave any room. Most of them have court dates coming up, where a judge will decide if they should go home, be sent to a group home, sent back to juvenile hall or sent "upstate" to do several years' time. Some of the youth here are innocent, picked up because they were in the wrong place at the wrong time. Other kids are incarcerated for continuously skipping school, or for robbery or murder. Several youth I see each week are there for murders they committed at fourteen or fifteen years of age.

In many ways the benefits of meditation and yoga for this population are clear. Many have learned no other way of dealing with stress than to act out in anger or seek "relief" through illicit drugs. While incarcerated, they are under enormous pressure from the system and other kids inside. Many kids are here for small nonviolent crimes, but become angrier and more violent while they are in the facility. They also spend a good amount of time by themselves in their rooms, when it is just them and their minds.

Contemplative practices give them another way of working with the stress they feel, and maybe more importantly, a tool for looking into their mind and heart to see if there is not an inner strength that is present, even amidst the great external turmoil. Almost weekly, I'll have a new kid in class look at me surprised after a meditation and say, "Wow. I felt high." Or after yoga they might say, "I've never felt like this before." I then talk about the power to be both relaxed and alert in any situation. Many of them have felt this while playing basketball or other sports. They know what it is like to be in the "flow" or "the zone."

When I introduce contemplative practices to them, I tell them that in some ways this is something that they already do. "What is the difference between 'chilling' and meditation?" I sometimes ask. Rather than introduce yoga and meditation as something new and strange, maybe it can be a more formal way of helping them do what they already do. I ask them, "What is the opposite of chill?" Most of the kids respond with the word "hyped." As best I can make out, it means to be anxious and stressed. I then ask, "Would people rather be chill or hyped?" Everyone agrees that people would rather be chill. So this is our common ground, our common denominator – no matter our age or skin colour. How can we help each other reach this goal? And how do we live in a way that creates less pain, both for ourselves and others?

With Michael, I know that if I try to convince him that what I have to offer is useful, I'll get nowhere. There is something else he wants to know – about life, about meaning, about love. He wants to know whether it is worth it to believe in anything. This is not something I can convince him of in words, only in the way I carry myself and relate to him. As my teacher used to say, "You can't really know the truth, you can only be it." It is this being or living the truth that the youth look for; the words you use are secondary.

How I relate to the guard as I enter the centre is as important as whatever I say in the class. The same is true with how I relate to the other staff and to the kids who are not into the practices. A number of months ago a kid named Jamal used to come to my class every week. Although he showed up each week, he never really tried to do the yoga, and during the meditation he would keep his eyes open and look around like he was bored. However, after the class he always gave me a big hug and said thank you. I later learned that he was on trial for a gang-related murder. I started to get frustrated with Jamal because I thought, "Why keep coming to this class if you are not interested in the meditation or yoga? What's your problem?"

It then hit me one day: he didn't come to the class for meditation or yoga; he came for a hug. He did not have the problem. I did. It might be the only hug he got all week. If he was not being disruptive, why not let him come to the class for a hug? I began to see how limited my views were of how love should be expressed. Gradually, Jamal was able to close his eyes for a short time during the meditation, and he seemed a little more engaged in the yoga. But if my devotion was strictly on youth doing meditation or yoga, I would have given up on Jamal a long time ago. I began to see how I could use anything, even meditation or yoga, as another thing for the kids to feel hard on themselves about instead of an expression of care and compassion for themselves. While certain guidelines need to be followed in class and I sometimes ask disruptive youth to leave, they need to feel a genuine care from me or nothing is going to work. If my care and devotion is not on them as people, then I'm just one other person with an agenda for them, one other person trying to fix them, and they want no part of it.

As someone who went through a great deal of pain as a teen, I remember that first moment when the world seemed to get bigger, when something opened. I certainly still had pain and difficulty, but something else emerged. While I cannot magically wave a wand and make everything better for these youth, I can help create an environment where the possibility of opening and healing is ever so slightly more possible. As a wise person once said, "Enlightenment is an accident; we practise to become accident prone."

Michael has since come back to a number of classes and has become one of the most engaged and curious students. The other day I asked him why he gave me such a hard time that first class. He looked at me, then dropped his head a little. "I had just gotten some bad news that day," he said, "and I just wanted to give someone a hard time. Sorry." I then realized that I often have no idea what the kids may be going through when they give me a hard time. Yet no matter what is happening, I create a space that does not attempt to force change or growth, but makes room for it to happen. This is a space that allows everyone to be just as they are – tough, afraid, happy, angry. Although the scene may look a little strange from the outside – a tall, skinny white guy who grew up in the plains of West Texas sitting in a circle of young kids of colour, mainly from the inner cities of New York City – there is a desire for happiness and well-being that we share. Our hearts speak the same language. So my job is not to save or to change people, but to help provide a space where compassion and wisdom have a slightly better chance of sneaking into all of our lives. ॐ

What do I *want* is very misleading. Ask instead, What do I think *my* life is *about*? Am I living in the way that I feel called, that I feel drawn, that I feel moved, that I feel inspired? Those are the relevant questions to me.

First published in Issue 11, Community, Fall 2001

opening to the unknown
the courage to live in community

[Bo Lozoff interviewed by Soren Gordhamer]

b o Lozoff has never been a traditional kind of guy. Coming of age in the sixties, Bo and his wife Sita were counter-society young people of that era – travelers, adventurers, hippies, activists. Later this calling led them to more formally structured spiritual practices such as meditation and yoga, and to living a simple life in an ashram. Both Bo and Sita quickly saw the joys of community life, and realized that a life focused on satisfying their needs rather than their wants was inherently more satisfying. As Bo puts it, "We could see that everything beyond shelter, weather and food is just gravy."

With the pull to service growing stronger in him, and after many visits to a relative doing time in prisons, Bo and Sita saw the similarities between the lifestyle they were living in the ashram – no movies, TV, sex, social life or drugs – and the life of prisoners. With the help and support of Ram Dass, the Prison-Ashram project was born, and little did they know at the time where this one idea would lead. The project has now become a worldwide organization that has helped countless prisoners. Their work involves mailing free copies of Bo's books (*We're All Doing Time, Lineage and Other Stories*, and *Deep and Simple*) to thousands of prisoners, corresponding and providing spiritual support to those inside, and giving talks at prisons throughout the country. They also invite prisoners to come stay at their community after they are released, and one former prisoner has now become a central part of the organization. In Bo's recent book, *It's a Meaningful Life: It Just Takes Practice* (Viking Penguin, 2000) he directs his teachings to the general population and gives a profound look at what it means to live a meaningful life in our day and age.

About seven years ago, Bo and Sita took on a new experiment: the Kindness House, an intentional spiritual community in North Carolina where people from all walks of life come to live simply and do the Karma Yoga that runs the organization. Bo has said that, initially, it was not easy leaving his home with Sita to start an intentional community, but something stronger was calling him to provide a place where both former prisoners and karma yogis could come live together and serve the greater good.

Bo was one of the main inspirations for me and my friend Andrew Getz to start our own nonprofit, The Lineage Project, which works with incarcerated teens. In fact, we got our name from the title of his book of short stories, *Lineage and Other Stories*. From my interactions with Bo over the years, I knew that in our interview he would not just say what he thought people wanted to hear or what would be popular. Due to this focus, I have not always found Bo to be the "easiest" person to talk to, but he is one of the people from whom I have learned the most. I was lucky to catch Bo right before he was embarking on a year in silence, starting with a forty-day retreat in a small cabin. In this interview, however, Bo has a great deal to say about the benefits and challenges of community life.

Soren Gordhamer   There have obviously been many rewards from your work at the Kindness House, but what have been some of the difficulties of community life?

Bo Lozoff Any ashram is going to have an enormous amount of difficulties because ashrams and communities draw people who are looking for an easier way, where everything is always going to be nice for them and they don't have to challenge themselves. And of course, any true spiritual community is exactly the opposite. You come into a spiritual community and everything begins confronting you, your frailties and your weaknesses and your vanity and your arrogance and your ego. A true spiritual community is a place where you go to annihilate your ego, not to fulfill it.

So ironically, and poignantly, I'd say the great majority of people who are drawn to a spiritual community are people who aren't right for it at all. They're looking for an easier way, and it's a harder way. It's easier, spiritually, to be out there living as a nuclear unit. You have freedom of choice, your own vehicle, your own income. If somebody says, "I've just never been able to hack it in that dog-eat-dog world," we just know they're not going to hack it here either.

The difficulties have been many. I don't know of another ashram or community that deals with the community we deal with. We have convicted killers coming here after twenty-five years' imprisonment, and we have college students coming for an internship and a retired schoolteacher coming. So it's a mix of populations, and it's been challenging. Kindness House has been around for a little over seven years now, and we've gone through probably hundreds of people who thought they wanted to live here. Right now we have a group of about fifteen very harmonious, mature spiritual people who have made an informed choice of why they want to be here.

And the fifteen of us live and work here as a family. It is NOT egalitarian, it is NOT a democracy. I want to be emphatic about that. It is a spiritual community. I am the director. We have a board of directors over the whole organization. Because it's our nature, we try to empower people to take responsibility, but we are not really interested in what people want. We assume that people who want to live here already have a good feeling for the flavour of the Human Kindness Foundation and the general drift of committed personal practice and committed service. We assume that people understand that there is no one right way to run a community. There are many reasonably good ways, and we have one of them. And we make it clear when people come that we're not really interested in their immediate contributions to making this a better place. They need to learn how to be the new kid on the block, do things exactly as we do without saying, "This might be a better way." We ask people to not make suggestions for the first three months, because we find that most people do not last three months.

SG So they are being asked to trust the community and trust the people who have been there longer.

BL   Yes, and trust is an enormous factor when you're in community, especially spiritual community. Somebody the other day asked, "How is your daily work schedule made? How are decisions made?" It's hard to answer those questions, because the whole thing just flows so fluidly. Decisions are more of a recognition than a few people who coordinate things. If someone doesn't have trust, they won't last more than a few months. If there is trust, there will be true consensus. None of us cares more about the object of a decision than we care about the process of each other making that decision.

When we have our board meetings every couple of months we remind ourselves at the beginning of the meeting that we are *not* here to make decisions. We are here to collectively intuit where God wants us to go next with the Foundation. We're here to collectively intuit what our guidance is, rather than knocking heads to make decisions. So our decisions are always consensus. And it's not a formal consensus like I've done in some other groups; it's just effortless, it's natural. All of us know that when there starts to be a little bloodshed in the discussion, that we're missing the point. When the object becomes more important than the process, we say, "Wait, what's happening here?" Last year we bought fifty-five more acres of land. That's a big decision. And we had disagreements. At some point one of us has to be insightful enough to remind everyone to take a moment of silence. We all know that we don't want to just get what we want, we want to come from a deeper place. And then we'll quiet down and come back at it from a different angle. It's a recognition rather than a decision. And that's our consensus.

That process takes an enormous amount of trust and intimacy. Everybody who's come here from prison, at one time or another, has said they'd rather be in prison than here. Everybody who's come here from prison has said that this is harder than prison. And I'm talking about people who have been raped, people who have been brutalized, people who have seen their cellmates killed over a pack of cigarettes. They have come to Kindness House and said, "This is harder than it ever was in prison." Every single one of them. Dozens.

SG   What do they mean by that?

BL   I think in a true spiritual community, you have to open into a trust of not knowing. In prison it's exactly the opposite. You are totally responsible for figuring out your own survival, what you need spiritually and practically. Although prison life is very difficult and you may be completely unsupported and you don't have any other resources to draw on, at least you understand the decisions you're making.

SG   What does the community do to maintain harmony?

BL   We have meetings every Friday night, we call them tunings. It's like tuning a guitar. You have six different strings on a guitar, and they can sound pretty awful with each other, or they can all be different and sound in harmony. We try to look at whatever's come up and really be open and communicate. We remind ourselves of what it is that we really want here and what we're doing here. It's not always to respect each others' boundaries; it's not to interact with each other in a way that always makes you feel good.

Sometimes I feel like the whole American spiritual community has been taken over by psychological or psycho-emotional pampering of each other. There's an attitude of "Oh, sorry, I don't want to say anything to upset you." Well, why not? I'm on this train to the end of the line, I'm not just trying to make the ride comfortable. There's somewhere we're going with all this. So we try to look at things like that in the tunings. As well as open up and say what's bothering us, like "so and so said something to me…" And you know the vast majority of the times, it's misperceptions and misunderstandings. When you bring it up in open communication the other person says, "Oh, I'm sorry, I didn't mean it that way at all!" And you say, "Oh, well, gee, I'm glad I said it."

The two main community practices are Karma Yoga and goodwill. What we mean by Karma Yoga is that every job merits equal respect and equal mindfulness and capability. That there's absolutely no difference to us between writing the books and washing the dishes. And that it's not a matter of what I like doing and what I don't like doing. You don't come to a place like this to talk about what you enjoy and what you don't enjoy, because we are able to enjoy any task that needs to be done. We are able to see it as God's work. And the goodwill practice is simply that we do not justify a resentful, angry feeling toward another. We may naturally have them, and experience them, but when we do, there's some spiritual work to do to regain the goodwill between us. The square one of goodwill is that we're all good people and don't mean each other any harm.

SG   I know that a lot of people, particularly in mainstream society, want more of a sense of community in their lives, but they're not quite in the place to move to a spiritual community. What do you think these people can do that might help bring a sense of community into their daily lives?

BL   To be really truthful with you, I feel it's very difficult to bring much sense of community into the typical nuclear kind of mainstream life. That lifestyle is a *brutal* consumer of time and resources. Internal resources as well as external resources. To pay all of your own bills, to have all of your insurance, and to maintain your vehicle and do your shopping and cleaning and cooking. For each person or small family to do that by themselves is just brutal. I just spoke with a woman last night who lives in Indiana, who said, "I work a forty-hour-a-week job, and there's just no time for anything else. Between getting there, getting back, doing my shopping, doing my cleaning, I don't know how to do other volunteer work, I don't know how to have a community."

We all pay for what we get. If we want the freedom to have all of that personal choice stuff, then you have to be willing to give up some of the pros of living in a community with people. Here, if a car breaks down, it's not one person's stress. It's just a car, and there's usually somebody who's the one to wind up taking it to get fixed. So it doesn't destroy your whole day. If you want community like that, you have to be willing to accept that you don't just hop in the car and go ten miles to Dairy Queen just because you feel like having a cone. We have to pay a price for what we want.

I think people who live in the mainstream sometimes pay too high a price. They would really love most of the benefits of living in a community with others, but they are just not willing to give up their freedom. "I want to eat what I want, when I want." At Kindness House, we do not eat between meals, period.

And for some people that's like, man, why are you so rigid, why are you so institutionalized? We're not institutionalized, we live on alms. We don't feel that it's proper to just open up the refrigerator because you've got a little bored energy. People support us to do the work that we do. And so we try to be respectful of that. And we don't feel that it's a lack of freedom, but I can understand how somebody else could. And so you give up a lot of freedom to be in community. Or, you give up a lot of the community benefits to get your "I wants." You just can't have it both ways.

SG   Do you feel that by serving as an example of how community life could look that you are helping others move toward more of a community life?

BL   We receive hundreds of visitors throughout the course of a year. I feel like there's certainly an interest and curiosity among many people to visit communities and to get a taste. A lot of times, it's somebody who's been on our mailing list for a long time and they're directly curious about us. But a lot of times it's just people who are doing tours of communities and they want to come and spend a few days in this one. And I think that's a great idea. I think that people who have done that have really opened their eyes a lot. They've had a chance to talk with many community members and have seen a lot of misconceptions about community life. That's one thing that people can do, is simply take a little time to go and visit different kinds of communities. Even if it's not a community they think they'd ever want to live in. It's always educational to visit communities.

SG   Is there anything else that you could say to someone who's living their life and maybe feeling isolated, or lacking a connection with people throughout the day? What guidance would you have?

BL   Just acknowledging the situation that we're in is helpful. We are in the most isolated era of human history. We have pseudo-connections through things like email and the internet. But there's never a human touch. You don't see a face. People don't have to even go to stores anymore. It's easier to just go online and buy it. So I feel that by first acknowledging that we're in a massively lonesome and isolated period, then at least we have sympathy for our position.

And then we can say, "I need to address this in some way, and how do I do that?" You can read an appropriate book, you begin to take measures, you try to do some volunteer work, or you look up some communities, or you read an article like this one, and you say, "I think I'm going to go try to spend a few days at that place." Just to feel it, just to see. You know, we don't want everybody in the world to try to move to Kindness House, because we have hundreds of visitors a year; we don't have room for all those people. But after they visit, people can go back to where they live, and they look with new eyes, because we ask people to ask themselves the real questions. "What is it that my life is really about? And how does my daily life jive with that? If I were to die today, would it be perfectly okay because I know that I've really lived the way that I felt moved to live?" And you notice I'm saying things like felt *moved* to live, and what is life *about*, rather than, What do I *want*? What do I want is very misleading. Ask instead, What do I think *my* life is *about*? Am I living in a way that I feel called, that I feel drawn, that I feel moved, that I feel inspired? Those are the relevant questions to me.

SG   How do you live out these questions at this point in your life?

BL   I'm trying to feel a very present, very real energy, an intelligent force that is moving me along on a path. And if I can get in sync with that force, then the whole world is my community, the whole place is my ashram. If I'm not in sync with that force, I could be at Kindness House for fifty years and feel isolated. So wherever we are, I feel like the work is always the same. Whether it's in community, or out of community. Do we still believe, like all the sages have told us, that life is about moving beyond the small, petty self? Or, have we changed our minds? Do we feel like the small petty self is actually really cool, and we want to work with it, satisfy it? I think that's the crossroads that contemporary culture is at. Deciding what do we really believe in? And is it worth it? And depending on what we say we believe in, is it worth a measure of sacrifice?

I'm going into a deep retreat in September. I'm going into forty days where I'm basically presenting everything that I have been holding on to, for total ego death, for total ego annihilation. I really don't care to come out of that little cabin forty days later unscathed. I would like to either be carried out in a body bag, or come out really significantly different than I went in. For me it's down to, What do I believe in? What do I believe in? And I find that I really honestly do believe in ego annihilation for the benefit of all beings.

Tukaram, the fifteenth-century saint, said, "The death of the ego is a festive occasion beyond compare." I really believe that, and so I'm going to present myself, saying, let's do it. I'm not holding out to see my unborn grandchildren, I'm not holding out for fifty years of marriage, I'm not holding out for watching more prisoners get saved or helped. This is it. Bo's putting all of his chips in the centre of the table. Whatever the next stage is, let's do it. And I think that's all that any of us can do when we feel isolated, when we feel like we need more of a sense of community. You can just open up the door and you don't have any guarantees of what's through it, but you know that where you're coming from is no longer satisfactory to you. And so you go in open. Leave behind what you know is not touching you in the deepest core. And don't worry about what lies ahead, but just be willing to leave that other thing behind. Walk into the darkness. ॐ

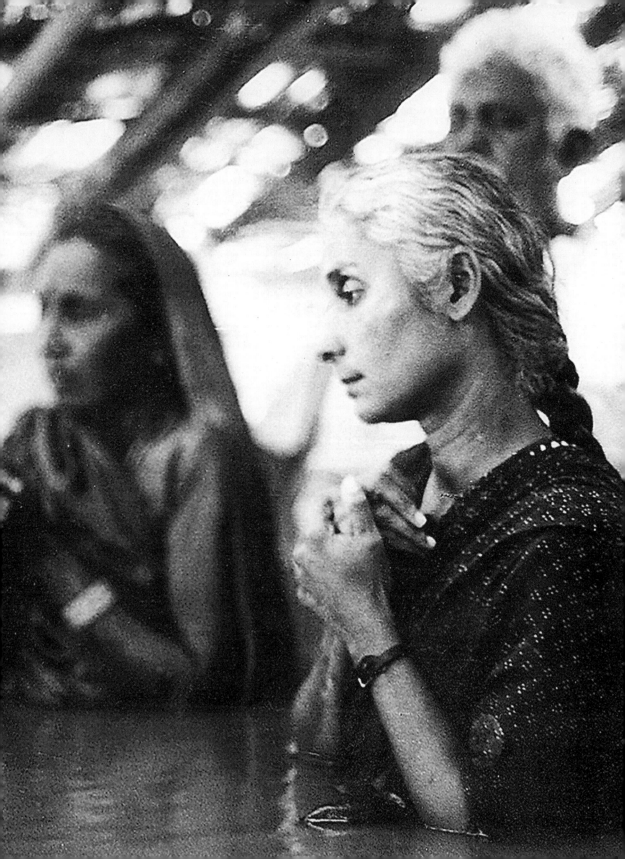

First published in Issue 9, Environment, Spring 2001

valley of tigers

the struggle over the narmada river

[Arundhati Roy interviewed by Swami Sivananda]

it is not much wonder that water becomes such a strong focus for development. It is the basis of survival. The planet has only a fixed amount of water; it is, in essence, a nonrenewable resource. It is easy to take for granted, to waste and pollute, when you have it. But when you don't, as increasing numbers of the world's population are discovering, water becomes like liquid gold. We can't live without it.

Damming and diverting rivers, harnessing water that otherwise "wastes away to the sea," is often seen as the epitome of re-engineering nature for human benefit. Irrigation and power projects are commonly thought of as synonymous with increased food production or clean and cheap energy. These projects have become an almost unquestioned foundation for prosperity around the world.

Over recent decades these water projects have become bigger and bigger. Now it is not uncommon for huge areas to be flooded behind dams. Entire ecosystems are submerged. Hundreds of thousands of people, often indigenous or subsistence

photo by Harikrishna & Deepa Jani

and farming families, are routinely displaced. All this has been viewed as the price of progress, necessary for the greater common good. But this is changing.

In 1991–92 I was the environmental advisor to the independent review requested by the president of the World Bank to examine the Sardar Sarovar Project being built on the Narmada River in northwestern India. The review was headed by the retired head of the United Nations Development Program, Bradford Morse, and the respected Canadian jurist, Thomas Berger. What has become known as the Morse Report documents an alarming discrepancy between what India and the World Bank said they were doing in the name of "development" and what was actually happening because of Sardar Sarovar. The Bank withdrew from the project in 1993. Then India's Supreme Court halted construction.

But the Narmada controversy continues to simmer. In 2000 it came to a boil, again. In a controversial split decision India's Supreme Court allowed the Sardar Sarovar construction to recommence. Shortly afterward, in London, Nelson Mandala released the report of the World Commission on Dams, calling for a whole new approach to the assessment of costs and benefits of these mega-projects. And upstream on the Narmada, the next project, the huge Maheshwar dam in the state of Madhya Pradesh, began moving closer to construction on a business-as-usual basis. In January 2001, 8000 people took to the streets in protest. And so it continues.

The Narmada is a holy river, Siva's river. Lord Siva is that aspect of the Hindu Trinity symbolizing the power of destruction. Siva is the remover of all obstacles. It is ironic that what is being proposed for the Narmada is the largest water resources development project in the world, a multi-billion dollar, basin-wide scheme affecting three states with the construction of 30 major, 135 medium and 3000 minor projects. Along with the dam, the project entails construction of some 75,000 kilometres of canals, cutting through thousands of small farms. The decades-long confrontation involves all levels of government, the police, the army and the judiciary. It includes international development agencies, multinational engineering companies and financing institutions, and environmental and human rights organizations in India and around the world. In some ways it is all befitting of Siva himself.

An inside view of what is unfolding can be seen through work being done by two women – Medha Patkar, a catalytic force in the protest movement in the

Narmada Valley, and Arundhati Roy, India's Booker Prize–winning author of *The God of Small Things*. In 1991, in the village of Manibeli just upstream of the Sardar Sarovar dam site, I sat with Medha Patkar on the steps of the Siva Temple in an all-night meeting as villagers poured out their concerns about what was being done to them in the name of progress. That village and temple have long since been submerged in the backwater created by the first phase of construction of Sardar Sarovar. Recently it was all brought back to mind when I heard of the galvanizing effect of two essays on development published by Arundhati Roy. In her small book, *The Greater Common Good*, she writes about the Narmada issue in language so clear that it cuts right through the comfortable clutter of economic rationalizations, engineering justifications, legal arguments and political rhetoric we have created to bolster our assumptions of what "develop" means. Through Arundhati Roy, the project-affected peoples of the Narmada have found their voice. A long-held belief, a whole worldview, is being shaken anew from New Delhi to Washington.

The decades of unquestioned water mega-development projects seem to be coming to an end. Why? The answer comes in response to astonishingly simple questions: Who benefits? Who pays? and How? These questions originate not in public or private sector boardrooms. They come from the valleys and villages where those people reside who are being asked to sacrifice what they have, in many cases who they are, all in the name of progress. In India, on the Narmada River, people are now saying no; they will not move. They are taking a stand, demanding nothing short of a new accounting for, and a new definition of, development.

Swami Sivananda   Why would a writer like you be attracted to an issue like the Narmada Valley?

Arundhati Roy   Initially, since I didn't know all that I know now about it, the attraction was a very instinctive one. The idea of people fighting to save a river was something that I am instinctively attracted to, since, you know from my book, *The God of Small Things*, my life was spent on the banks of a river in Kerila. For writers not to understand these issues is something that suits the people who build these dams very well because it's a world of technical mumbo-jumbo and nobody really knows what's happening. Everyone's eyes glaze over. It is only a writer of literature, and a writer who is read, who can insist on writing about it in a way that people who don't know anything about this issue can understand. When you get to understand what's really happening, then you realize that you just can't be sitting around writing sweet short stories to address these issues.

SWS   For people who wouldn't be familiar with the Narmada, how would you summarize what you see happening there?

AR   The story of the Narmada Valley is the story, not just of modern India, but of what is happening all over the world. The Sardar Sarovar Project, the first dam on the Narmada, is displacing close to half a million people, half of whom are not counted as "project affected" in order to make the project sound viable. For fifteen years this dam has been under construction. They haven't managed to resettle even one village according to the directives of the Tribunal, which says that villages should be resettled as communities. For fifteen years people have been fighting. From there you begin to inquire into the role of big dams. Why is this country so committed to them? What is really going on? Are they really the temples of modern India, as Nehru characterized them?

The figures that you come up with are just so shocking. First of all, shocking because there aren't any government figures. But then when you actually keep at it what emerges is hard to believe. India is the third largest dam builder in the world. These dams have displaced 56 million people. We don't have a national rehabilitation policy. We're told that dams are the key to India's food security, but they say that only 10 percent of India's 200-million-ton food-grain produce is from big dams. And you know, 10 percent of all the food that India produces is eaten every year by rats! So what are we doing?

SWS   So you are questioning the whole notion of progress?

AR   Exactly! How do you measure progress if you don't know what the benefits are and what the costs are? Is it an article of faith? Progress for whom? Even the way progress is quantified by planners is absurd. It is quantified by how much you consume. So, India has "developed" because today it consumes 20 times more electricity than it did in 1947. But they don't tell you that still 80 percent of rural households don't have electricity. So, just because a smaller section consumes a lot more, India has developed. One would imagine that these are pointers in the opposite direction.

SWS   When I was in India I often heard, particularly from World Bank and government officials, that this kind of development is something that people in the West had long ago embraced and India was just following suit. The notion is that this is the price of progress.

AR   Yes. This is what I hear every day of my life in Delhi – that someone has to pay the price for development and that the "voluntary forced displacement" of 56 million people is the price tag. But I have a very crude and simple analogy for this. If you were to say, okay, because somebody has to pay the price, the government has decided to freeze the bank accounts of 10,000 of India's richest industrialists and citizens and distribute their money for the "greater common good," can you imagine what would happen? So I think that these ideas roll very easily out of the mouths of people who are not involved in paying that price.

SWS   Didn't the government of India and the World Bank both have policies that were exemplary in many respects on resettlement and on environmental matters? Are they saying one thing and doing another?

AR   It's an unwritten agreement, not just in India, but in the whole business of the World Bank, that you make these humane-sounding, consummately written policies understanding that they will never be implemented, and that the people they are written about will never see them or hear about them. In fact, one of the things I'm writing now is how as a writer one spends one's life trying to journey to the heart of language and use language to express thought. These officials are engaged in the *exact* opposite enterprise, which is to use language to mask their intent. They use language to say things that sound politically correct and perfectly poised in their morality. But it has nothing to do with what is happening on the ground. That is understood! A study was recently released in India that showed that 90 percent of all the river valley projects have just completely broken their environmental guidelines.

SWS   Where do we go with these insights, insights that are now becoming more and more common not only in India but all over the world? We seem to have caught the theme of what's wrong, but what happens now? What is the option here?

AR   I think that the option is a really simple one, but very complicated at the same time. The option to greed is less greed. I see it so clearly. It's really just a question of using a *little bit* of wisdom and having some respect for other people's lives. It would save so much of the world. I don't think that everybody in the world is an evil-intentioned person. But they don't understand what the connection is between switching on their light and what happens in a river and what happens to the people who live on the banks. And scaling down the lifestyle without being a Gandhi or becoming a hermit or going around in loincloth – I don't think you need to do that. I think you could still live a wonderful life and yet have some respect for what you're doing.

Instead, people, especially American companies, are here goading us into the privatization of power in order to play, as they say, in the twenty-first century. Their solution for hunger is to increase the appetites of the well-fed. It is lunatic. It makes no sense at all.

SWS   The people in the Narmada Valley, in these villages, how do they see what you're doing?

AR   The only time in my life I've felt anything akin to "national pride," because I'm not a nationalist and I don't believe in country, is when I go to the valley and see the spirit of the fight. I really think this is the spirit of this country. All over the world, other such fights have been squashed and people have been shot and broken. But here it goes on. And, to me, one of the reasons that it goes on is that the alliances are so wonderful. The movement is often criticized. The people in the Narmada Bachao Andolan [Save the Narmada Movement] are criticized for being outsiders but I think that's precisely the strength of the movement. Where you have these alliances being made – between urban and rural, between writer and farmer, between painter and fisherman, between student and boatman – that is what gives it its strength and its rigour.

My essay ["The Greater Common Good"] has been published in the local languages, so those who have read it know what I'm saying. For those who haven't, or can't read, they just know that I'm sort of a famous person who said quite simply and unequivocally that "I'm on your side," and I'm not trying to sound like some reasonable intellectual. I recognize that this is a war and that you take sides. The people know that their voice has to be carried outside the valley, and they know that I'm one of the people who is doing that.

SWS With your work, and the leadership of Medha Patkar, it looks as if women are playing an important role in the Narmada Valley movement.

AR   Yes, in the Narmada Valley, especially in the Maheshwar area, you have to just come to see what the women are doing! It is unbelievable. Just tigers! It's a valley full of tigers. The women in the villages are *so* ferocious. It's fantastic to watch, to be involved in something like that. I think that women are the future now. Some time has passed since we've unshackled our minds, and that energy is phenomenal. It's going to change so much of the way the world is and thinks it ought to be. The fight to save a river is also a fight against the notion of a destroyed world. I think women are not as crudely aggressive, and the fight to save something fires our imagination more than the fight to destroy something.

SWS In the end, what does saving the Narmada Valley look like to you? What is the outcome?

AR   I think that we are fighting specific wars in specific ways. And if the world were to join together to save the Narmada Valley, it would be a first step toward saving much more. It would be a victory for *so* much else. It would be a victory, to begin with, for nonviolence, which is one of the most wonderful things about that fight – nobody has picked up a gun, yet. And it is a fight of such magic and such imagination. The only thing, the *only* thing worth globalizing is dissent. To allow this fight to be crushed will be a defeat for more than the Narmada Valley. ॐ

[UPDATE: The construction of large dams on the River Narmada in central India and its impact on millions of people living in the river valley has become one of the most important social issues in contemporary India.

Arundhati Roy continues to be concerned about what is going on in the Narmada Valley. In July 2004, she visited the valley of Harsud town in Madhya Pradesh when submergence was imminent. She wrote "Road to Harsud" which was published by Outlook *magazine (www.outlookindia.com).*

The struggle on the ground continues in Gujarat, Madhya Pradesh and Maharashtra. It is due to the struggle that further destruction in the valley has been delayed as of now. However, thousands of families affected by the massive flooding have yet to be resettled. Many peoples' movements representing the poor and underprivileged continue to fight and protest in order to stop destruction due to the proposed and ongoing dam projects.]

They are just boys,
I think, as I stand
there between rows,
tiptoeing around legs
and sprawling arms,
unclenching fists,
straightening necks.
Young men who wake
each day just wanting
to love and be loved,
like us all.

First published in Issue 16, Social Action, Winter 2002

sahodaran

as the HIV pandemic escalates, what can transform the fear and ignorance that sustain it? friendship.

[by Michael McColly]

arriving in India feels like coming into a cosmic war. There's an initial revulsion, an instinctual recoil of your body as it is bombarded by the chaos and cacophony of too many souls trapped in one place clamouring to escape. Dead bodies float through the streets on the shoulders of men; Bollywood dancers spin and sing from TVs in tea stalls; Divine utterances spray over the city from gaudy temple tops and Islamic spires; three-wheeling diesel rickshaws, taxis, buses and thousands of motorbikes spew clouds of fumes into visible heat; masses migrate from village to city, from city back to village; the rich, the middle class, the poor and the poorest of the poor swarm in the streets, moving from tinted-glass software complexes to squalid squatter shacks made of mud and thatch.

Despite the painful realities of this schizophrenic nation of many peoples under one flag, I feel oddly at ease here – even at home. I first traveled to India five years ago, and it was here that I learned my body itself would teach me how to live with HIV. I spent two months in Mysore studying yoga. I remember nothing could have prevented me from doing so, not the nightmares I had of getting sick and being admitted to Indian hospitals, nor the warnings from doctors. I needed to come to India to not only face the fear of traveling with HIV, but to also face what was ultimately behind every diagnosis – the fear of death. And yoga became my lifeline, the only thing I could trust in those difficult years before and after I was diagnosed. Yoga kept me sane and safe.

When I returned to Chicago, I began teaching yoga to others with HIV, which led me to South Africa to attend the International AIDS conference and offer a workshop on the benefits of yoga. Being among activists and teaching others with HIV demanded that I embody more deeply the healing and transformative nature of yoga. A year ago I sold my belongings and left my teaching post, determined to tell the story of how those around the world are transforming themselves as they transform their communities – despite the fear and ignorance that sustains this pandemic.

This pursuit has brought me back to India, and as I arrive in Chennai, a city exploding under the weight of too many people and too few resources, my teacher will not be an aged guru, but activists, doctors, sex workers, and those like me who live with HIV.

I am on my way to meet a man named Sunil Menon who works in AIDS prevention with both sex workers and men who have sex with other men, MSMs, as they are termed in AIDS parlance. Western terms such as "gay" don't apply to the kind of situational cultural conditions of South Asia when some men may choose to have sex with other men because they have no other sexual outlets in a society such as India where premarital sex is taboo.

As my taxi pulls to the curb in a tree-lined street of Chennai, the dark-haired, cherubic-faced Menon appears, scoffs at the price of my taxi, grabs half of what I am about to fork over, pays the driver, and with a theatrical flourish escorts me up to a second-storey flat into the cramped three rooms of Sahodaran.

Inside, young men sit at a table and flick wooden plugs about a board game, two more attend phones at desks, others mill about socializing. Upon my entry, hands quickly go through thick waves of shimmering black hair, shirts are straightened, pants dusted. One by one they approach my sweat-soaked shaggy self, offering their hands, nodding, staring directly into my eyes with daring confidence.

Sahodaran ("friendship" in the South Indian language of Tamil) is an organization that promotes community development and safer sex practices for these young men. Started in 1998 by the London-based Naz Foundation, Sahodaran addresses the growing sexual health crisis among males who have sex with other males since the rise in cases of HIV and other STDs. Sahodaran aims to establish a community among these generally uneducated and poor young men by training and educating them on the risks of HIV/AIDS. The "boys," as Menon fondly refers to them, even though most of them are in their twenties, are trained on how to advocate for safer sex practices by handing out condoms and introducing Sahodaran to men whom they meet on the streets.

"They have no place safe to socialize, to be themselves without getting teased or hurt," Menon explains with a sigh. "Most days I can't get them to leave when I go home." A doctor comes once a month and provides basic care, and if they choose they can be tested. However, many don't choose to do so. They don't want to find out, knowing that if word gets out of their positive status they will no longer be able to work. Menon hopes that in the future they can provide job training for the young men – computer skills, English, tailoring – but funds, of course, are scarce and just having a little food and tea on hand for them eats up the tiny budget.

Out of a back office emerges Shivananda Khan, Naz's director from London, in jeans and a black shirt, with equally black hair. Computer printout in hand, Khan's attitude is all business, fierce and passionate, matching his lionlike face. He sizes me up, tilts his head and listens when I blurt out who I am and that I'm there because I want to write about the lives and work of activists who are HIV positive. He nods. "You taking the cocktail – yes?" It's the question that I know I will have to face many times in the next several weeks – a fact that is almost harder to say than admitting my status, as it underscores the vast difference between those who have access to treatment and those who don't.

"I got to get a cigarette or I'll go crazy," Khan jokes as he goes out the door, but then pauses and turns back. "D'you mind if I reveal your status to the boys? They need to meet people like you." He turns to Menon and nods my way. "Let's get Michael to talk to them."

"Sure, sure," I say, eager to please, but not knowing what this might really mean.

Khan has helped to set up other programs like this one for MSMs in several other Indian cities as well as in Pakistan and Bangladesh. He is the activist's activist, summing up the situation in India for me with a sarcasm that could only come from one who'd been seasoned by his third decade of deaths and governmental indifference to the rights and health of South Asian men who, like him, do not conform to either the narrow moralistic illusions about sexuality held by Indians nor to those Western models that misidentify MSMs as "gay."

Menon gathers the boys so that Khan can go over a few things and do a demonstration on condom use that they can duplicate in the field.

Khan's voice is passionate, belying a deep sadness in his eyes. He knows the odds that these young men face and the risks they pose for other men as well as women – most of these young men are either married or will be. Like everywhere in the world, HIV/AIDS has become a disease of the young. He implores them to trust one another and make this community work. "You have to take responsibility for yourself and each other. Who is going to look out for you? The police?" The boys all laugh.

"Look," he says, with Menon interpreting into Tamil, "we're all at risk in here." And to my surprise he points to me. "Ask our friend here from America how easy you can get it." Suddenly twenty pairs of eyes are scrutinizing my body, trying to find that hint of illness. "How many people know someone who has died of AIDS?" he asks. All hands go up.

Tonight our destination is Chennai's beach, where thousands of the city's poor come each night to escape the heat, amble among the makeshift stalls that sell food and trinkets, and mingle in the darkness. I've come with Menon and Gunaseelan, one of the fieldworkers. The beach is a prime cruising spot and so this is where fieldworkers hand out condoms as well as meet their clients if they need the money. The rickshaw driver drops us off. It's growing dark. I can't see where I'm going, but follow dutifully.

We hike up and down mounds of sand, through dry weeds and trash; rats scurry and hop; men move in and out behind trees. A man pops out from behind a clump of bushes by a miasmic little pond. Gunaseelan greets him and they walk back into the shadows. Menon and I follow at a distance. I have gotten to know Gunaseelan in my visits at Sahodaran. He might be twenty but looks much younger, and as I watch him disappear into the darkness, I feel a little nervous for him, seeing now the world in which he works. But there he is opening his satchel to hand some condoms to the man, who then returns back into the bushes.

By now it is dark yet still steamy. I can see the glow of lanterns and hear the din of an invisible mass of people. But the only way I know I'm on a beach is that it's difficult to walk in the trash-strewn sand with my sandals. Finally I can hear the surf and children playing and begin to see clusters of people, sitting on their haunches eating. Closer to the lanterns, I see them now, their bony bodies, their handsome thin noses, their gleaming oily black hair, their dark eyes peering out of pools of pure white, their shirts unbuttoned and flapping in the breeze from the sea. They study me, too, the blond man from America with the smiling teeth and the anxious body. We amble up to a long line of vendors that fans out onto the beach. We pass wooden tables with vats of sauce and rice, women frying chapati, pastel-coloured candies in glass boxes, tea in tin urns, sweaty bottles of Coca Cola, biscuits stacked in plastic jars.

I see that we have drawn some attention. At first I think it's me, but no, it's me with them, the feminized men Indians call *kothies*. "They all know what these boys do," Menon whispers to me, pointing to a couple of guys selling sodas who smile knowingly at us.

I buy everyone sodas and offer to take pictures. Combs come out and they begin to tuck in shirts and primp, using each other as mirrors.

Walking back to catch a taxi, couples and young people stroll under the large banyan trees next to the dimly lit street. As we stand by a bus stop, three women come scurrying toward us, waving, bangles jangling, silk scarves flowing off their necks. But when they approach, I'm suspicious. Nose rings, gaudy faces, diamond *bindis* don't quite camouflage their maleness upon closer inspection. The fieldworkers and Menon greet them with hugs. I offer my hand and they giggle, nervously. They are the *hijras,* transgendered males, hermaphrodites or neutered men who from ancient times are sanctioned by Hindu tradition for ceremonial purposes at certain temples. Harshly ostracized, they are mistrusted and seen as a sign of bad luck if crossed in the streets. Thus, custom has it that you must give them money if they ask or else suffer their evil will. They run off now, skittish, fearful of being seen by the police who frequently beat and rob them, as they do the fieldworkers, blackmailing them for sex as well.

As I look back toward the beach into the blur of the lantern lights, the colours and sounds mercifully wash out the harshness of the city before me. I marvel at the human instinct toward romance. By the Bay of Bengal on a beach strewn with litter and shit, one still finds the brightest saris, the diamond *bindis* between the eyes, the sugary sweets, the mirrors framed in seashells, the photo galleries where one can put an arm around a cardboard Bollywood star.

I see these young men roving about under the bushes and think how pathetic and painful to be reduced to performing these humiliations, but being with them in their world they remind me of the power of human affection and where it comes from. Affection, itself, our yearning as awkward as it is toward the Divine, never fails us. What is cruel is not what these young men must do to survive, but that in our ignorance and fear we determine what affection is and who shall have the right of its embrace.

In India, for most of those with HIV, it's a slow, agonizing and humiliating death. Despite the fact that India's own pharmaceutical giant, Cipla, now manufactures copies of the effective antiviral drugs and sells them in India and throughout the developing world, they are still too expensive for most Indians. In fact, it's still very difficult to even find doctors bold enough to see HIV/AIDS patients, let alone treat them. But in Chennai, thanks to Dr. Suniti Solomon and other doctors at YRG Centre for AIDS Research, who reported India's first case of HIV back in 1986, there is now one lone clinic in all of South India for people with HIV and AIDS.

When I arrive, I find women doing laundry and spreading green bedding on weeds outside a two-storey renovated building set off from an aging, well-used public hospital. Inside I walk by patients clustered in corners, mostly men, thin and weary after traveling sometimes as far as 200 or 300 kilometres to see one of the four doctors who practise there.

Although there are twelve beds, YRG mostly serves outpatients. Those who are too sick either die at home or are brought to the government TB hospital, an overcrowded embarrassment that Menon warned me against visiting: "Don't go there, Michael. The patients are dying on the floors and hallways. Why would you want to see this?"

Waiting for one of the doctors, YRG's office manager and social worker, Ms. Sunita, offers me tea and suggests I talk to a regular patient, who volunteers to sit with new patients, particularly women. I sit in a small freshly painted yellow room and in comes a beautiful, petite woman not more than twenty years old, in a scarlet sari with a canary silk scarf. She is shy at first, her hands folded, held tightly to her chest. I watch her face as the social worker interprets in Tamil. I can tell the exact moment when the patient learns of my status, as her head lifts and she looks into my eyes. I nod, held by her naked stare. Her voice becomes excited and I scribble furiously. As her story pours out in Tamil, her body becomes more and more animated, until it feels as if she has taken up the entire room.

She tells me her husband, a lorry driver, infected her. And upon his death, and the death of one of her children, she discovers she too has the virus. Instead of finding solace in her family, her mother-in-law throws her out of the house, accusing her of infecting her son. Thus she is left practically homeless. One of the many ironies of this very typical story of AIDS in India is that infidelity is almost unheard of among married Indian women. Remarkably, she is healthy, which she attributes to YRG and to a group of women like her with HIV. She smiles when describing this group, known as Positive Women's Network, which according to Sunita is the only family she has. Groups like hers provide child care, share food and work on collective income-generating projects, but most of all, they offer each other desperately needed emotional support. "She knows she will die," Sunita tells me, "but she is not afraid now…because she knows these women will raise her daughter."

One of the doctors is now free, but before I leave, I ask if she has anything to ask me. With her radiance she studies me, and then turns to Sunita and speaks. "She wants your card if you have one and…she wants to know…" Sunita pauses, thinking of how to phrase the question, "she wants to know if you have a group like she does – or someone – who takes care of you in Chicago?"

I fumble, stalling, looking for my card in my shoulder bag. Embarrassed, I don't know what to say. I have no group. No "someone." I say something about friends and family and smile with that smile I use when I am not quite telling the truth.

The doctors are harried and worn, not just with the ever increasing patient load, twenty-five to thirty a day, but the endless international officials, doctors and press that make demands. I'm worried that I'm doing the same, but they are intrigued that I have come, a writer with HIV without an affiliation, and like the good doctors that they are, the first thing out of their mouths is a series of questions about my own health, concerned that Chennai might be wearing me down. And when I admit that I haven't eaten lunch, I'm commanded into a back office behind a curtain to share their lunch of curry and rice.

"Why haven't you called?" Menon's voice is a mixture of disappointment and relief when I return his call from my hotel. "The boys keep asking me, 'When is Michael coming back to teach yoga?'"

After the evening on the beach, I spilled out my story in all of its dark details of how I'd contracted the virus in ways not so dissimilar from the casual sexual lives of the fieldworkers. It wasn't so much their bold questions about sex or confusion about how I could look so good if I was sick that made it so difficult for me. No, it was having to face them alone, having to look at them as people, not as a statistic or a photograph in a magazine or interesting anecdote to bring back to America, but as real young men who needed more than a pep talk from a whiny white guy. Or was it that by having to talk with them I had to face myself? Later that night, a familiar sadness came over me in my hotel room. I drank two tall bottles of head-splitting Kingfishers and lost myself in what seemed like an endless stream of beautiful Indian women who danced across my television until I fell asleep. I was exhausted and knew how much energy it took being around them, so I had to take some time. But I hadn't forgotten my promise to teach them some yoga.

When I arrive at Sahodaran my anxieties vanish into the vibrating atmosphere of a room full of young men eager to know where I've been and if I'd brought back the photos I'd taken of them on my last visit. Their hunger is seductive and somehow assuring.

We crowd into a small back room. We can barely close the door and Menon has to exclude more than half of the boys, literally pushing them back and closing the door, promising that he will show them the poses later. We have no mats. They aren't wearing appropriate clothes. Most can't understand much English. "Take off your socks and lie down." I tell them through one of the boys whom Menon chooses as a translator. "Close your eyes and listen…listen to your breath," I say, wondering whether this will work at all. They fidget, fix their shirts, jostle, clown and whisper with one another. I take a deep breath myself.

I ask them to follow my count as they inhale and exhale. It helps. As I count and they breathe, the room quiets, the whirr of the air conditioner meshes with the street sounds below and I begin to take note of their bodies. Sympathetically, the rhythm of their breathing brings us all together.

After a few minutes of silence, I ask them to open their eyes and come to a sitting position. I see individual faces, softened eyes, and looks of disorientation. We do a few poses on the floor – I'm winging it, watching them and thinking what to do next.

We do Camel pose: they lean back, some grabbing ankles, chests lifting; and then I tell them to fold down into a Child's pose, stretching their torsos and arms out in front of them on the floor. Going around the room, stepping over bodies, I gently press down on their backs to lengthen their spines. And as soon as I touch them, feel the bones of their back through their shirts, I know why I am there. I need them as much as they need me.

They stand. We try full Sun Salutations, but confusion reigns. I stop them. "Let me demonstrate. Watch me."

I do a simple Sun Salutation, right leg back, arms up, left leg back, Stick, Cobra, Down Dog, etc. The look on their faces almost makes me laugh. Total confusion. "Just follow me, *Suryanamaskar*," I say, suddenly remembering where I am and thinking that using Sanskrit might help them.

"*Suryanamaskar, Suryanamaskar*," I hear them whisper to each other, smiling openly at me, as if I'd finally figured something out, as if the name itself is the pose and all those complicated movements only something you do if you don't understand the word. As I watch them, smiling uncontrollably myself, it dawns on me, that it is the name, the word itself – *Suryanamaskar* – that has brought us together. The first pose we all learn. The one I recall learning in an acting class in college in the seventies. From my first visit to India I recall that children are often taught this pose by their teachers or at home by their fathers. I have to stop them finally as they seem to be like wind-up dolls set in motion and unable to stop.

We do more standing poses and I use all the Sanskrit I can effectively pronounce. "*Virabhadrasana!*" I stick out my arm and bend my knees. They follow, relishing our new relationship, as tenuous as it is with my poor command of Sanskrit. I hold them in Warrior pose, wanting them to feel it, adjusting arms and legs. They strain, eager to please me. I am moved by their sincerity, their yearning bodies, desperate it seems to fulfill this image of the warrior-hero.

Yoga, the ancient discipline of the Brahmins and priests, has now become ironically the new trend among the Westernized elite and educated class in

Mumbai and Delhi. How absurd, I think, *teaching yoga in India to Indians*. Or is it the absurdity of modern India itself – a nation that exports grain while its people starve; a state that honours the ethical wisdom of its founder Gandhi, only to hold on to beliefs that deny basic human rights to women and people of lower castes; a sophisticated society that educates hundreds of thousands of engineers and scientists to create a technological and economic boom for only the West to exploit.

As we continue the more challenging poses, I see some wither from lack of stamina and no doubt from lack of food as well, but for most I see that shimmer in the eyes, that brightness in the face, that quickening of the body that is Yoga.

I try to help them where I can to feel the pose, pulling back shoulders, planting feet, massaging necks. At first, they feel fragile – tending to tighten or recoil when I touch them, but as we reach the end and the Corpse pose, they sigh and seem to spill out onto the hard tile floor. And as they let me press and pull and soothe, they expel their own tenderness into me.

They are just boys, I think, as I stand there between rows, tiptoeing around legs and sprawling arms, unclenching fists, straightening necks. Boys, yes, who I can't help seeing in other poses behind bushes, in the darkness of alleys, and along rivers, but young men just the same, who wake each day wanting to love and be loved, like us all.

Afterward they line up to offer me their gratitude, shaking hands, bowing, the bold hugging and kissing me on the cheek. And then one boy comes up, eyes a blur and full of emotion, grabbing me as if I am a mirage he's finally been able to catch: "Oh, Sir. Thank you. Thank you! I never do this before." And before I can respond, he's wrestling with the door and his emotions as he bursts out of the room, pushes through the throng of other boys, and runs back into the street. ॐ

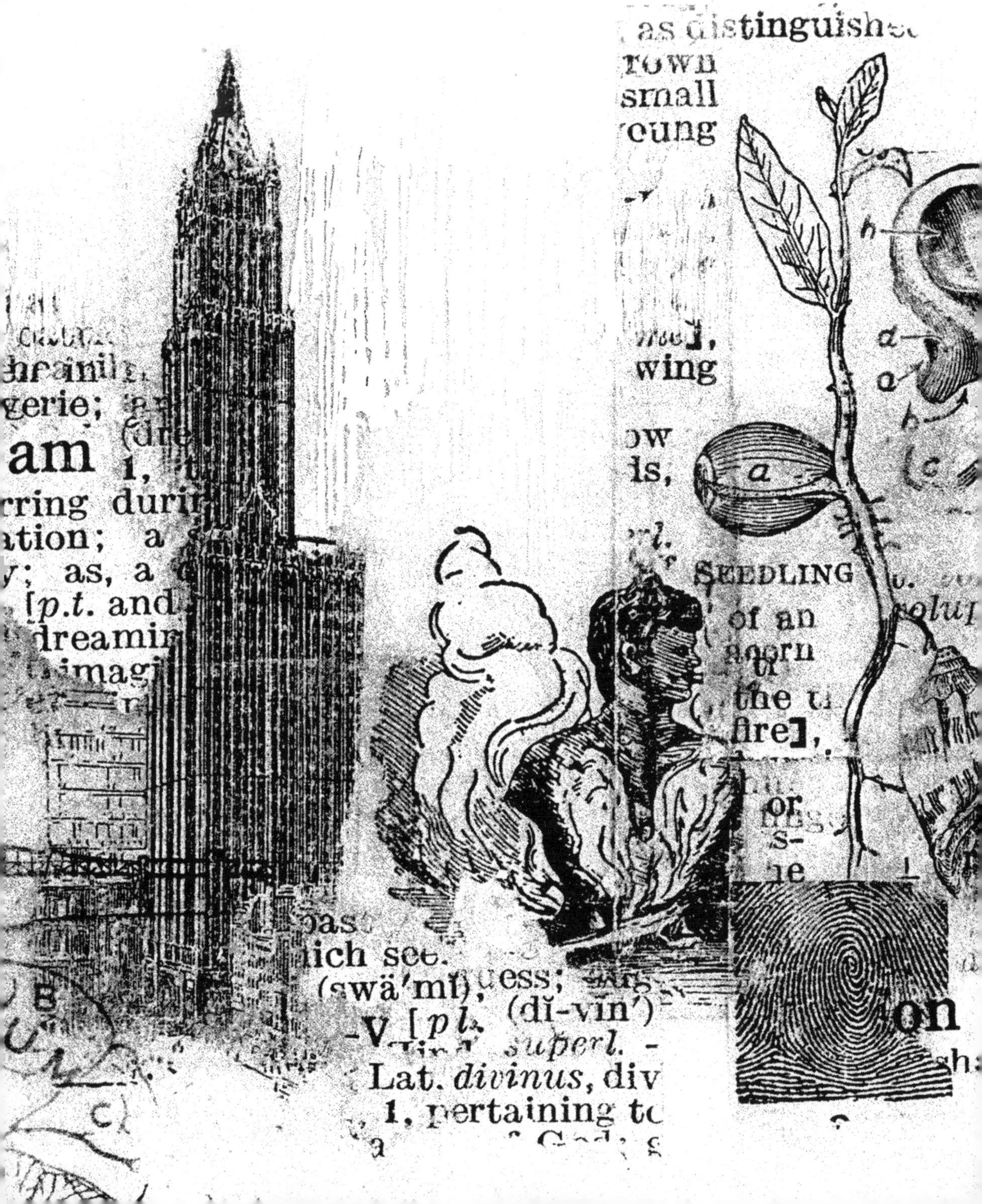

as distinguished

rown

small

oung

wing

ow
ls,

SEEDLING

of an

acorn

the u

fire],

or
s-
le

am

dreami
imagi

ring durin
ation; a
y; as, a
[p.t. and
dreamin

ich see.
(swä'mf),uess;
-V [pl. (di-vin')
superl. -
Lat. divinus, div
1, pertaining to

on

First published in Issue 19, Myth & Storytelling, Fall 2003

theory into practice

what is the future of yoga?

[Georg Feuerstein interviewed by Swami Gopalananda]

georg Feuerstein is passionate about the yoga tradition, which he calls "...a spiritual wealth too valuable to discard." Building a bridge to that spiritual wealth is what his life's work is all about. He's written many books on the subject, including a new one: *The Deeper Dimension of Yoga: Theory and Practice,* published by Shambhala. Reading it, one cannot help but be amazed by the awesome spectrum of yoga philosophy and practices available to us. But even so, the questions remain: Are these ancient traditions of yoga relevant to us today? And if they are, how do we find the real thing?

A researcher who loves his subject, Georg is often dismayed by what passes for yoga in the marketplace, and he cites the example of the Tantra tradition, which has been identified in the West as the yoga of sex. "Nothing could be further from the truth," he says. "From the outset, Tantra understood itself as a 'new-age' teaching intended for the *kali-yuga,* the dark age of moral and

illustration by Cristina Sitja Rubio

spiritual decline." He goes on to say that "…Tantra offered new rituals, and gave philosophical ideas a new look and feel." He's describing a revolution in spiritual teaching that reached its peak a thousand years ago, but he could just as easily be describing what is happening in yoga today.

It is estimated that over 30 million people in the West regularly practise yoga as part of their daily routine. Inevitably, we are redefining yoga in our own terms, though the resulting practices sometimes seem far removed from their original intent. So where do the traditional teachings of yoga come in? Is tradition standing in the way of a "new" spiritual revolution? I put these questions to Georg in a recent conversation, and I came away from our talk inspired and hopeful about the future of yoga.

Swami Gopalananda   In the preface of your new book, you describe yourself as one who has for over thirty years been a champion of traditional yoga. What do you mean by traditional yoga?

Georg Feuerstein   Authentic yoga, as it has been taught in India. A spiritual tradition rather than what we have here in the West, which is a watered-down version of what people consider yoga.

SWG   How was yoga traditionally taught?

GF   Well, being an esoteric tradition, yoga has always been transmitted by word of mouth and through initiation by a qualified teacher. I don't want to denigrate Western efforts, spiritual efforts in the field of yoga – but in the West we have many so-called lineages that are secondary. In other words, some fifty years ago somebody read a book on yoga or went to a lecture by a yogi, started their own yoga practice, and then started initiating or communicating yoga to others. To me, that's not really authentic. I think very few Westerners are qualified to communicate yoga, first because they did not receive it from a qualified, authentic teacher. Second, because in this part of the world we by and large ignore the great merit of studying the thing that we teach. So we make it up as we go along. But study has always been a central part of the yogic tradition.

SWG   How do we build a bridge from the traditional roots of yoga to what is happening today, where millions of people are practising yoga, and yoga studios are popping up everywhere?

GF   This is exactly what I have been trying to do by introducing these deeper aspects of yoga through the medium of study. By studying, people at least know what yoga is and hopefully get intrigued enough to go out and look for teachers who can convey authentic yoga to them.

There is an external side to yoga and an internal side. The internal side is what's largely missing. So we have a lot of *technique,* especially in Hatha Yoga. But we don't have very much internal communication, which is the essence of yoga, which is given in the process of transmission from teacher to disciple. So we consider ourselves students of yoga, very much in the Western model of a student and not necessarily as a disciple, a disciple who takes on the discipline given by the teacher.

SWG   When you refer to the internal yoga as the "essence of yoga," can you tell me what it is you're describing?

GF   Let's take *asana* practice, for example. A teacher can show you how to do *Savasana.* In other words, lie on your back and relax. But the inner experience is what makes it a yogic practice. Very few people, and I have observed many students, know what this inner process is unless they have had instruction by a qualified teacher. And the great mystery of yoga, of course, is this transmission. And it's always amazing to me how a person who hasn't had that kind of exposure to the inner side, the transmission side of yoga, can actually go out there and teach meditation, for example. It doesn't work. And so we find after years and years that people finally admit, well, it's not working for them. They're sitting there and watching themselves think, and they're bored, and they give up.

SWG   You said earlier that our Western idea of study is very different from the study you are talking about here.

GF   Right. In yoga, it is called *svadhyaya,* which means literally "one's own (*sva*) going into (*adhyaya*)." So it's "one's own going into something," or we can have a second interpretation, which is "one's going into oneself." And study in the yogic sense involves both. It is studying a subject in a meditative way where we kind of wrap ourselves around it. And at the same time we are aware of our own process, the study of ourselves, which is missing in the Western education system.

SWG   You are saying that we have a situation where there are very few qualified or authentic teachers, which leaves us wondering: How do we find what you're talking about? What is the way?

GF   Well, in my case I went to a teacher.

SWG   How did you know the teacher was authentic?

GF   That's the great mystery. I think it's a matter of how desperate you are for Light. And you go for that; you look for it. When I was in my late teens I found a teacher. He was an Indian and had his school in Germany at the time. I saw his picture in a health food store, and I knew this was the teacher I would be studying with.

From then on, it was always a play between receiving teachings from qualified teachers, and then internalizing all of that, processing it and integrating it through my continued practice and study of the texts. In studying these texts, you encounter a wisdom, a quality of mind and heart, that can strike you and make a difference in your own feeling and thinking. For myself, there isn't a day when I don't pick up some text and be inspired by it. It's always a signal for the mind. Once the ground has been prepared, it doesn't take very much to go back on track if we stray from our understanding of the process and the awareness that it cultivates.

SWG   And preparation of the ground means what?

GF   Preparation of the ground means that we are always ready to examine ourselves, and to remember whatever teachings we have been given by a teacher. Now many people, of course, don't have access to a teacher. Often I'm asked, you know, How can I find my guru? And I always have to laugh because my experience has been the guru really finds you. And that you simply prepare, prepare, prepare for that eventuality. And even if it never happens, the effort you have made, as the Bhagavad Gita reminds us, is never wasted. Whatever effort we make to grow inwardly, whatever effort we make to increase our understanding and cultivate the virtues that yoga tells us are desirable virtues – such as non-harming, non-stealing and truthfulness – whatever effort we make to cultivate those, all of it will sit within us and it's the only thing we are going to take when we leave this Earth.

The teaching is the primary vehicle by which we learn. Even if we go to a teacher, we need to have our focus on that. If we are fortunate enough to have a teacher who strikes us so deeply at the level of the heart and beyond that we can make this required gesture, in the traditional sense of yoga, of self-surrender, then we must do that. And the benefits of surrender have been demonstrated throughout the ages in the yoga tradition. People wake up.

SWG   What does it mean to "wake up"?

GF   Waking up simply means that we get in touch with who we are beyond the body-mind, and that this great wisdom the teachers manifest is going to manifest in us as well. My process has always been a very gradual one. There's so much we can do and learn prior to all these elevated states of mind and transmission and whatnot. Really, it is up to us to realize that we are in a fix. In traditional terms, we are suffering. So how can we get out of the suffering? We have to do something about it, and that's where the traditions come in, where the teachings of sages can tell us something.

SWG   There are many great myths associated with the ancient tradition of yoga. What relevance do they have to us in the West today?

GF   There are some people who respond to symbols and metaphors and images more than others, and then there are those who have an obstacle perhaps to Eastern or, specifically, to Indian symbolism. My own sense is that unless we are sensitive to symbols it is very difficult for us to relate to *any* spiritual teaching. Part of our psyche has to be activated. It's the softer side of our mind. It's like we have to become artists in the process of our inner growth. In fact, as we grow, that side of the mind becomes more prominent. We see things differently. We enjoy the fact that there are images and symbols that trigger in us this deep process of transformation.

SWG   You're talking here about a part of the mind that is not so rooted in the reasoning or intellect, but in the intuitions and feelings.

GF   Yes, the creative part of the mind. The imagination. We all access that part of the mind, of course, in our dreams, but the fact that we don't value our dreams and those images is an expression of our disinterest in that aspect of the mind altogether. So in yoga, the interest is activated. Part of the yogic process is that we become sensitized to our hidden nature, or the subtle body or subtle realms. We touch them in our dreams, but we must also touch them in our waking state.

SWG   There's a kind of irony in this. It seems you're describing a side of mind that is more feminine or receptive in nature. But in the tradition of yoga, and it seems to be happening in the West, too, is that the "name" teachers, so to speak, are usually male and the tradition is largely defined by men. Where is the feminine side in the teachings and why is that not coming forward in the teachers who are defining yoga in the West today?

GF   Well, the way I would look at this is that the yoga tradition has survived largely through its literature. That literature was authored by men. But that gives us only one side of the picture of the history of yoga. My belief is, and I have no proof of it, but my belief is that yoga was taught just as much by women. In fact, we have an inkling of that in the Tantric tradition, that the early teachers were women, not men. And the only difference is that men have always wanted to rationalize everything, and so they were the ones who wrote the books. Women tended to do their teaching in a quiet, hidden way, and it's only some of them who wrote or whose teachings were written down by students that we know of.

In Tantra more than any other tradition, the feminine side is given great attention through the concept of Shakti, goddess power. You talked of irony. To me, the irony today is that we have so many male teachers, but the body of students is about 75 percent women. So my hope for the future of yoga rests with them! I think as more women become involved in the transmission of yogic teachings, we will see a different quality, and it will be the kind of quality that is very much integral to authentic yoga. You know, where do we get this interest in virtues? It's the feminine principle of the psyche. Men, I think because of their biological constitution and the kind of social experience they've had in recent history, tend to emphasize other values, such as competition. And that is a quality that is not found in traditional yoga. So we are at a difficult time. On the one hand, we have received all these teachings, and on the other perhaps we are not quite ready to practise them as they should be practised.

SWG   When you look at the mythology of yoga, can you see the seeds of the way yoga should be practised in the future?

GF   Yes. Tantra, to me, especially in its formulation of Kashmiri Shaivism and Mantrayana Buddhism, is a practice, a yogic tradition that has a lot to teach us. Tantra is the most sophisticated formulation of yoga, and I think it teaches us that integration must happen at all levels. Tantra was based on a complete re-evaluation of embodiment – the human body – and even the social system. Many of the Tantric teachers completely supported the notion that the female gender has the same, equivalent value to the male embodiment. And in fact, many of them even placed it higher, because it is a transformative embodiment. And if we allow the images of Tantra to impact on us, they can communicate something very profound about the spiritual dimension.

SWG   Can you give me an example of what you mean?

GF   One of the things that many students have a hard time with are the fierce deities, as in Buddhism – the protective deities like Mahakala, surrounded by a ring of flames and looking really fierce. Now if your reaction is so strong that you don't inquire into the meaning of this image, you have lost out. If you made enough room in your mind to accommodate something unusual, something different, then you can learn from it. So an image like that when we are open to it can really teach us about the fierceness of life, the "bloody tooth" of nature. Often we don't want to know about that, and so our society ignores or wants to shove aside death, sickness, all these things. But they are with us, they are part of life, whether it looks bad or it looks good, it doesn't matter.

SWG   You're saying that when we look at an image like Mahakala, we're really looking at a reflection of our own mind?

GF   Absolutely.

For me, all yogic myths are about our own mind. You know, the yogis had no interest in just telling stories. They told stories because people in those days worked more with the imaginary, intuitive part of the mind, and what they wanted was to leave a deep impression on their listeners in terms of the unconscious imagery. And all of them, when you look at these stories, all of them are about transformation of a bad situation into a good one. They all start out with a mind that is confused, that is suffering, and the yogic teachings in various ways have to hit us very hard to be motivated to overcome our restrictions, our limitations. So, for example, an image like Durga killing demons is really us, our Higher Mind, say that courageous part in us, confronting these limitations. One limitation may be that we dislike authority as a matter of principle. So the limitation implies that we won't listen. If we can find images to which we can relate, then we might see the joke. We might see that we are actually excluding ourselves from a whole wonderful stream of life.

SWG   We come now to the essence of all yogic teachings, which is accepting and integrating all parts of ourselves. How do people confront those reflections of themselves and accept that, yes, that is part of me, too?

GF   People need to understand the job that is confronting them in yoga. It is to be present as Consciousness. Consciousness itself has no fear. It also has no one-sided attraction to anything. It simply is. When we remember that part of our nature, and do so as often as we can and perhaps one day continuously, life is joyful even when the bad presents itself. In part, we understand life as a play, which in Sanskrit is called the *lila* of the Divine, the sport of the Divine. And we find that what we overcome as our fears can become available as energy to do something constructive.

Say you fall ill. Now instead of worrying about it and fearing all kinds of consequences – the imagination takes over and it is a negative, constricting type of response that suppresses our natural joy and energy – instead of going into that, we laugh and in the open space see the real humour of our activity. Immediately, there is energy for the healing process. We can be constructive. Or we have a relationship that is difficult, say a person who is always bothering us in some way. Instead of fixating on the bother, we see that this person is a signal to us to overcome some negative emotional pattern. And in that way, we start realizing that this person is our greatest teacher. The Buddhists say your greatest enemy is your most wonderful teacher. Why? Because if we can see that, we liberate our own energy for the process of living.

SWG   Do you have a personal experience of liberation or dynamic transformation?

GF   After my first teacher, there were many years that I went out on my own, and tried to do this thing of self-transformation. I had also, for many years, been shepherded in my spiritual process by a Sufi master, Irina Tweedie, even though I had no real interest in Sufism. But she was very kind and took care of me. I was with her for fifteen years and would quite often go to her little apartment in London and just sit and chat. She was a truly great Sufi master. One day I went to her and said, "I have to ask you a rather silly question. We have been together so long. Are you my teacher?" And she literally fell over on her bed laughing. I said, "What is going on?!" She composed herself, and said to me, "Georg, you would never accept a woman as a teacher!" I remember being very upset with her! I said, "How can you say that?" But she insisted. Then, after a little bit, she added, "Your teacher is just around the corner. Don't worry."

And then, very shortly after that, everything unfolded rapidly, and indeed I ended up with a teacher. I habitually distrusted authority, and he was a very radical figure, whose teachings to me were very profound and challenged me in my self-woven nest of security. And I thought to myself, if I ever really want to get out of the corner that I have painted myself into, I need to make a gesture here. And it took a lot to do that because he was an overwhelming kind of authority. When I first saw him, I thought, Oh my God, What have I done? But something in me knew that I needed to go through that lesson and find the middle way between being receptive and not being slavishly clinging to authority, which doesn't work.

You see, yoga has universal principles involved. But it is for every person a unique process. We must encounter these universal principles of yoga and make them our own, and we can do that only through our own personality, our own system of symbols, and so on. So whatever we encounter in yoga must be translated into our own terms or it won't work.

SWG   So when you encountered this teacher in a male form, it could be said that this teacher was Durga in action.

GF   Yes…oh yes! He was completely Durga. Being with him was the hardest thing I ever did in my life. And yet it was the one thing that benefited me the most. But still I had to learn to walk my walk. The teachings I received and the direct demands made on me to change, really I'm – even after all these years – I'm more grateful now for how he taught me, how he served me.

SWG   It wouldn't be accurate to say that you're a traditionalist for tradition's sake, but more that you feel tradition has a place in our lives today.

GF   Exactly. I'm a rebel by nature. As I said, I have a hard time with authority, a very hard time. But I can see the benefit of the wisdom of these masters. You know, their whole lives were dedicated to self-transformation, so what they came up with is worth listening to. And that is all I would hope people will do: take the time to listen. But, you know, if we don't have that capacity, we reject such a heritage of wisdom, 5000 years and more, perhaps. Why would we throw that away? Wisdom is not something you can discard. And we have so little wisdom today. Our society does not hand down wisdom; it hands down chaos. Our education system is not designed to liberate us; it's not designed to put us in touch with our inner happiness. On the contrary, there is no wisdom in it. That is why we need to listen to the traditional teachings.

SWG   Do you think we're in the throes of creating a new yogic tradition in the West, which at the moment is a little tumultuous and confusing?

GF   I think that is the best-case scenario, and I like to think of it that way. Jung, very perceptive man that he was, said that as the West is conquering the East through its technology, the East is conquering the West through its spiritual teachings. This is a remarkable perception, and I think it is a correct one. People sometimes ask me if I think it's possible that the yoga movement could die out in the West, but after a hundred years it seems unlikely. Increasingly, there is this wonderful flow between cultures and traditions. We are becoming one world, and the yogic heritage, the spiritual heritage will not only be part of it, but will play a very important role. There will be an emphasis on integration rather than specialization. And I believe also that future yoga will be a yoga that will be socially and politically engaged because that's part of our existence. We cannot deny that, and if we do, it will be equivalent to denying that we have a body.

SWG   *What I hear you saying is that in the yoga of today as it emerges into the West, we have the seeds for a radical transformation of how we live our lives together.*

GF   This is exactly my argument. How that will play out remains to be seen. In what I call the verticalist schools of yoga, the schools that are into world-negation and fleeing into the forest and so on, the world is played down along with the body, along with social action. This is no longer viable. It was never viable. I think that there are very rare individuals who can and should complete their inner process, their yogic process, away from everyone and everything. But they are very rare. It's like one in a billion, maybe! All of us are essentially householder yogins and yoginis, and we have to acknowledge that. We are involved in the world and we have not purified our karmic baggage to the point where we could happily, meaningfully, withdraw from everything. The work we need to do is not an inner separation from anyone and anything, but simply a physical separation – the space to do the work that needs to be done spiritually. Our job will be much more how to integrate all the different aspects and levels of our being, how to live in the world in a spiritual way. In yogic terms, we must learn more and more to be in touch with and to become who we are as Consciousness, and yet not forsake the other dimension of existence, which is in fact embodiment. ॐ

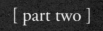

[part two]

inspiration / encounters with others

The subtitle of *ascent* magazine is *yoga for an inspired life*. *ascent* searches out yogis, often hidden, who have the gift to inspire. We all seek resonance with our own experience, we crave wisdom, we want to know about the sacred teachings that can open up our lives. Often a simple encounter, a moment, an action, becomes essential to our expanding experience of yoga.

Gem Salsberg writes, "I am so vast. I am so small. This is revealed to me by daily saints and common people living basic real lives. Practising compassion in their unassuming way and showing how essential it is to breathe and be grateful, love and be grateful, try and be grateful. The teachings of each day are modest and mostly silent."

What will spark an inquiry into spiritual life? Who guides us along on the path? There are inspirations everywhere, everywhere you look.

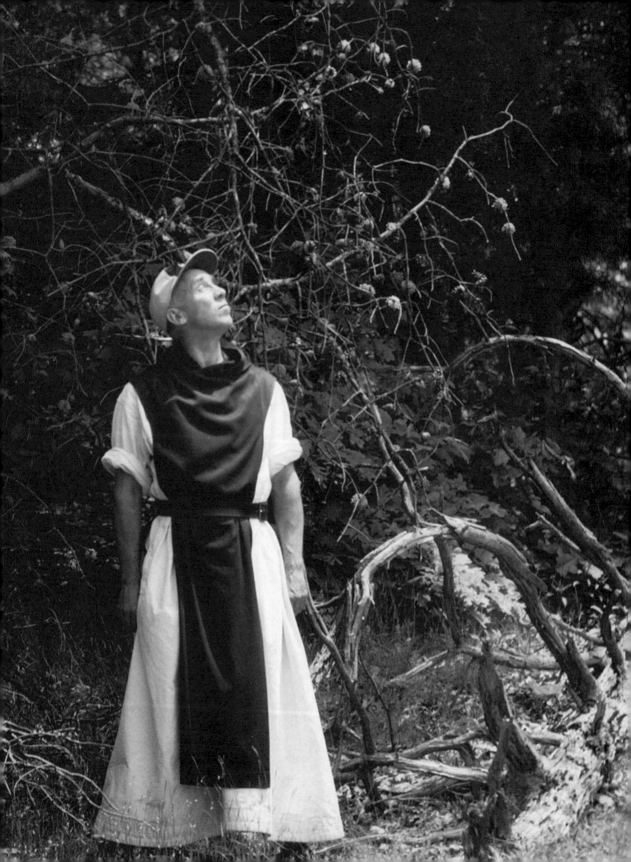

First published in Issue 15, East/West, Fall 2002

natural buddha
meeting thomas merton

[by Brent Burbridge]

in the sweltering heat of a Kentucky July, I stood in the midst of a hundred monks' graves. At the time, I didn't even know why I was standing among those small, perfectly aligned white crosses alongside Gethsemane Abbey; I only knew that the one we were all staring at read:

> Father Louis Merton
> d. December 8, 1968

Who was Louis Merton? Why would I visit his grave? In Buddhist philosophy, it is said that there are no accidents, but I didn't know anything of Buddhism at the time. Looking back, I can see I was meant to find this man, whom the pamphlet from the information centre called a saint, poet, essayist, monk, mystic and activist. It also called him Thomas Merton, his pre-monastic name. It pointed out that he had died in Bangkok while studying the religions of Asia.

photo © the Estate of Ralph Eugene Meatyard,
courtesy Fraenkel Gallery, San Francisco

Curious.

I hopped in the car twenty minutes later and sped off toward the Atlantic Ocean, having more or less forgotten Merton as quickly as I'd met him. The only remnant of this encounter was a small white and black prayer card on which was printed one of his meditations. A few lines made enough of an impact on me that I kept the card as a reminder. These lines were:

"…nor do I really know myself, and the fact that I think that I am following your [i.e., God's] will does not mean that I am actually doing so. But I believe that the desire to please you does in fact please you. And I hope I have that desire in all that I am doing."

These lines, more than the curiosity of a monk's graveyard, rattled around in my consciousness. They comforted me in a way few texts had before, since they ascribed higher value to my efforts to do God's will than to my final results. When it came to discerning the will of the Divine and becoming one with it, I was quite sure that neither I nor many others had hit the mark. It is what frustrates all of Christianity, to a greater or lesser extent – everyone is trying to hit the mark but few can agree on how.

I was brought up in a rather conservative Christian tradition concerned with doctrinal correctness. Understanding the will of God comes, for most Christians, through reading the Bible, interpreting its stories and instructions, then implementing them. To many it seems that implementing what one perceives to be the will of God can be fraught with error. I saw that many people either became overconfident in their vision ("I'm so right"), or religious neurotics ("I think I'm right…aren't I?"). No matter what, concern with "doing it right" is paramount.

What those lines of Merton's from the prayer card said was that there are not really categories like success or failure, accomplished or not accomplished – but instead, a will and a desire that inspire action. It is the spirit in which we act and our intentions that make us holy. I found this idea liberating; it opened up so many avenues of spiritual exploration and self-discovery without the fear of misinterpreting doctrine.

From the time I met Merton in that Kentucky heat – though I made no effort to remember him – he seemed to start following me around. Like learning a new word you've never heard before, which then begins appearing in everything you read, Merton began popping up everywhere. I'd see his books on shelves;

the priest would make a reference to him during a homily; favourite writers like Czeslaw Milosz would reference him in a poem or essay.

One day a friend suggested that we should choose a text to read and periodically meet for discussions over beer. Fine idea, I thought. "How about Thomas Merton's *Asian Journal?*" he asked. I declined, saying I knew very little of Buddhism, Hinduism or Asia in general. And I wasn't so sure about this Thomas Merton. I would be in over my head. I didn't know enough.

But my curiosity was piqued, and I picked up a copy of the book and began reading it in conjunction with Conze's *Buddhist Texts through the Ages.* A whole new mode of spirituality opened up to me, and as I sat in the sun skipping class I couldn't help laughing at myself for all the resistance I'd put up to this monk over the years.

Thomas Merton began as a thoroughly modern saint might be expected to: residence in several countries before the age of twenty, a humanistic education, Marxist dabblings, and a weakness for pretty girls and cold German beer. He had, since his graduate school days at Columbia University in New York, looked East for a level of inspiration that went beyond what literature and leftism offered.

While still a student, he attended lectures and seminars by a prominent yogi visiting from India. When Merton asked him by what texts he might find enlightenment (fully expecting titles from the Indian tradition), the yogi told him to start with the Western contemplatives like Meister Eckhart and Teresa of Avila. This stunned the young Merton, but he followed the yogi's advice. Just over two years later Thomas Merton took the vows of a Trappist, an order of reformed Benedictine monasticism, a form of spirituality at the very heart of the Western Catholic Christian tradition.

Yet Brother Louis, as he was renamed, never gave up considering the East a source of wisdom and technique that could inspire and revivify what he perceived to be a waning Western contemplative practice. In *The Asian Journal,* Merton writes that "by openness to Buddhism, to Hinduism and to those great Asian traditions we stand a wonderful chance of learning more about the potentiality of our own religion."

He felt this to such a degree that after years of studying Buddhism and Hinduism while practising as a Christian monk, he decided to travel to Asia.

He sincerely believed that there was not just the opportunity to learn more than books alone could provide, but to gauge first-hand what unity existed between the Asian traditions and Christianity. Bound for Bangkok, his flight rising above San Francisco Bay and then the utter blue of the Pacific's expanse, he wrote: "I am going home, home to where I have never been in this body." That home was the spiritual environment of India, Tibet, Bhutan, Thailand and Japan.

Merton's total openness to what all the ancient religions of Asia had to offer him, and their correlation to Christianity, is in stark contrast to my own story. I have always been very aware of other spiritual traditions and loved reading about their exotic beginnings, magical founders and inscrutable rituals. It was more of an academic exercise, though. "Don't get too close, because it's not what I believe to be true." That's what I told myself. What made me think that those Christian beliefs I then adhered to couldn't be added to, augmented, or cast in a new light? I was caught in the human desire for the known, for what is comfortable, for what one expects, even demands, to be true. Merton's example is of one who is so secure and confident in his own tradition that he is unafraid to go beyond it, into an unknown space.

In a spiritual context, yoga brings together the human and Divine, giving harmony to that relationship. The result is awareness of the world's true nature and liberation from it. The various types of yoga are different ways of achieving this end. Merton considered Christian meditation to be a yoga, in that it requires a calm, focused mind; it aims for total absorption into the object of its focus, which is Truth, whether you name it God or *samadhi*.

While Merton found a spiritual home in the East, I found one in his writings; as he sought further experience and knowledge of Eastern contemplative techniques in Zen and yogic traditions, I sought more of what I'd first read in those seminal lines from the prayer card: liberation – freedom from the absoluteness of doctrine and entry into a life of the spirit.

One of the many similarities Merton saw among spiritual traditions was encapsulated perfectly in the idea of Karma Yoga, represented in the West in the concept of Christ-likeness. Karma Yoga is "union with God in action," an integrated life of contemplation and action. As a monk, Merton knew of the balance of contemplative and active elements in life, and was often frustrated by their imbalance. It is a monk's job to pray. Merton sometimes chided himself for not doing enough about the things he prayed and wrote about. But prayer is doing, and actions are prayer, just as Krishna assures Arjuna in the Gita: "You must perform every action sacramentally." By acting and praying "sacramentally," Merton himself tells us, one avoids the "false affirmation of our individual self as ultimate and supreme."

Karma Yoga is in many ways a basic principle to understand, though often difficult to practise. It requires maintaining focus on a thought or task, or not being impeded by concerns extraneous to your task, such as what others will think or the accomplishment of pre-established goals. Karma Yoga is a spirit of action that I am still trying to understand and practise in my everyday life. In all things, I try to work from within for my own satisfaction, and the satisfaction of the Divine who has placed me here in this place at this time among these people. To live according to this spirit is a gift to both God and one's self.

One of Thomas Merton's critiques of the Western tradition was that people prayed to God that they might do His will, but were not open to all that might mean. In a word, people lacked selflessness. Monks and laypeople alike expected things to be a certain way, in essence expecting the Kingdom of God to take the form their own mind imagined it should take.

In Christianity the highest ideal is the *imitatio Christi*, the imitation of Christ, who was the selfless servant, whose every action was perfectly attuned to the Divine will, and devoid of individual aspiration or concern. Christ is almost a perfect argument for the truth of Buddhism, in that there are no categories, no oppositions, but complete unity and reconciliation in the Divine. Human and Divine are one. Self and God are one.

Merton understood this primarily in the Christian sense – that becoming one with the will of God leads to extinguishing of the self, like an individual flame that is absorbed into the fire. A biblical analogy is the Body of Christ. All believers are a part of the whole, the integrated body, with Christ and Christians bound up together in a perfect unity, to carry out the will of God in the world. Buddhism says that the cycle of birth and death, *samsara,* ends when the individual becomes perfectly absorbed into the fabric of the universe and self is extinguished.

Merton, so human in so many ways, reveals in his journals that he was very much an individual, and one of this world to be sure. But he had the striving. For he is constantly catching himself in self-absorption and determining that he will renew his struggle to set himself free. In this way he is so human and so holy at the same time.

I recall, some years before I began to read Merton, spending quiet evenings on a friend's rooftop, discussing our different spiritual paths. Her background was yoga and Buddhism; mine was Christianity. We were never adversarial, but I saw no way our ideas could be reconciled at the time. Like Merton's prayer card, which germinated something new and substantial, our conversations about yoga and meditation worked slowly within me, changing me from the inside out. Looking back, what must have seemed unremarkable events at the time seem now to be almost logical steps toward the opening of *The Asian Journal*'s pages. What seemed random was totally organic. It's true, I now tell myself, there are no accidents.

While journeying through Asia, Thomas Merton (Brother Louis) was given yet another name by a Tibetan lama: *rangjung Sangay,* or "natural Buddha." The lama's name was Chatral Rimpoche. He and Merton had spent several hours together talking about the mutually intriguing similarities between Buddhism and Christianity. Chatral had been meditating in solitude for over thirty years at his hermitage in the Himalayas, and within a few hours of Merton's company recognized a man of deep knowledge, compassion and devotion to the spirit.

Around the time of his meeting with Chatral, Merton wrote in his journal, "I want to be the best Buddhist I can be." Did this mean that his Christian faith was diminishing as his interest in Buddhism and other Eastern meditative traditions grew? No. For Thomas Merton, the two were already one; it only remained for him to bring his mind to such clarity, to such one-pointedness, that it might fully perceive the unity that already existed.

Near the time of his death, Thomas Merton addressed a group consisting of Christian and Buddhist monks gathered in Calcutta. As he stepped up to the podium he put aside his notes, declared that his clerical collar was really a "disguise" that he almost never wore, and began speaking to them directly from within. His final lines echo as vibrantly and with equal comfort for me as those first lines years ago in the Kentucky graveyard:

"My dear brothers, we are already one. But we imagine that we are not. What we have to recover is our original unity. What we have to be is what we already are." ॐ

Instead of using the word "renunciation" we call it a determination to be free. Renunciation often has such a negative connotation, but it is actually a very joyful spiritual aspiration.

First published in Issue 20, Renunciation, Winter 2003

determined to be free

brother wayne teasdale, thubten chodron & swami radhananda on renunciation

[roundtable conducted by Clea McDougall]

September 8th, 2003. I find myself talking with a swami, a monk and a Buddhist nun. I want to find some humour in this – there's got to be a joke you could tell – but really, I feel a little unsettled. Good unsettled. Unsettled in that way you feel when you are maybe a little dejected but then hope creeps in.

Here are three real people who have committed their lives to paths of renunciation. Bikshuni Thubten Chodron, an unassuming, clear and curious Buddhist nun; Swami Radhananda, our soft-spoken powerhouse of a columnist; and Brother Wayne Teasdale, an interesting mix of Christian monk/*sanyasi* making his way as an urban mystic.

I gather them together to dispel some of the myths around renunciation, to redefine renunciation for modern practitioners. Who isn't curious about the lifestyle of a monk? Who hasn't wanted to ask, what is it like for them? And how can we, who aren't quite ready for life as a swami, still practise renunciation?

The renunciates are from three very different traditions but they share an essential truth. Their words circle around each other, overlap and weave together a vision of spiritual commitment. What strikes me is how much they have been inspired by their own teachers, and how the commitment to spiritual life becomes a service to others, a way of giving back. Renunciates have a role beyond their own evolution; they act as symbols of the possibility in spiritual aspiration and intent. Their renunciation does not mean that they have turned away from life but that they fully engage in their true responsibilities to the world.

I have always wanted to do the total renunciation thing, and listening to them talk I feel moved by what they describe, but a little sad that I am where I am on this path. At the beginning.

September 8th happens to be an auspicious day for me. It's the anniversary of the mantra initiation my guru gave me eight years ago. This day is always one of questioning for me. I have to admit to sometimes indulging in despair about the state of modern practice and spirituality. How do I really live a spiritual life in the world today? How do I release my attachments? Is there hope for us? Is there hope for me? Talking to these three individuals today seems like a little message from the Divine to keep on, and even if I take little steps, there is hope.

I start off by jumping right in and asking: *What is this thing we call renunciation?*

Brother Wayne Teasdale It's really the renunciation of, or freedom from, what we would call in the Christian tradition the false self, the egoic consciousness, or the self-cherishing attitude. Leading up to that, as a monastic, there is renunciation of some of the usual joys and pleasures of this life, including owning property and having a family and things of that nature. But that's just the beginning of renunciation.

Swami Radhananda For me, renunciation is going toward something. As a renunciate, I have made a choice where I want to put my energy and how I want to live my life. It's knowing the teachings and then having the opportunity to share them with other people. The clearer I become on this path, the more that drops away. Also, I only take what I need. I let go, but at the same time other things come to me. So it's a real contradiction in some ways.

Bhikshuni Thubten Chodron   It's a determination to be free from cyclic existence with all of its unsatisfactory conditions, and an aspiration to attain to Liberation or full enlightenment. From a Buddhist perspective, we're renouncing suffering and the causes of suffering. I would suggest in a Buddhist way, instead of using the term "renunciation," we call it a determination to be free. Renunciation often has such a negative connotation, but it is actually a very joyful spiritual aspiration.

Clea McDougall   People often do react negatively to the idea of renunciation, and equate renunciation with selfishness. Is it a selfish choice?

WT   Of course it looks selfish to the world because people are conditioned by this culture where the basic focus is the nuclear family. In the Hindu tradition, and also in Buddhism, it's very common for someone to have an awakening and leave their wife or husband and children. And that, to Western sensibilities, is outrageous and looks incredibly selfish. This culture looks for a sense of permanency in life, but everything is impermanent. Renunciation is not negative; it's not a withdrawal from the world. It's withdrawal from the world's illusions, and from the whole selfish way of life, which is the basis of suffering.

And what I've come to is that renunciation is the condition for the possibility of entering the kingdom of heaven here. Jesus says the kingdom of heaven is in your midst. What does that possibly mean? The kingdom of heaven is the realization of the primacy of compassion, the primacy of charity, and that the whole of the world and all our relationships with all sentient beings is governed by this sense of caring, of concern, of kindness. To be able to realize that in each moment is being in the kingdom of heaven.

TC   We are renouncing suffering and its causes, and selfishness is included in the causes of suffering. Renunciation is going toward freedom from selfishness, so I find it very interesting that people see it as a selfish thing when our whole motivation is to free our mind from selfishness.

Where can we go in the world where we are not in relationship to others? Even if we live a more private life or more like a hermit, we still live in constant relationship to all living beings. And these contemplatives are more aware of the plight of all living beings. Many people who live in the city block everything out because they have too much on their plate. Renunciation isn't leaving our relationships with others, it's a way of transforming them.

From a spiritual viewpoint, our consumer society looks very selfish. People talk so much about my family, my career, my vacation. Even though those people are very busy and they're living in the world, that appears selfish.

SR   The other thing about selfishness is that a lot of people will take time out of their lives with a busy job, or to do a Ph.D., for example, and that takes a lot of time away from their families and focuses on something that is totally theirs. And this can be a good thing: the Ph.D. can nourish the mind; the job can help support the family. But sometimes they forget about their families, instead of drawing them in or making a more meaningful relationship with them. So you can do something for yourself, and also be aware and giving to those around you. It's a choice, whether you are a renunciate or not.

CM   So how can we turn around our definition of renunciation into something positive?

WT   It's embracing a fuller life. It's funny, there's a wonderful aphorism by Saint Erenaeus that says, "The glory of God is the human being fully alive." Fully alive to love and compassion and selflessness and kindness. Freedom from grasping of self and trying to fulfill one's individual pride and egoic notions of happiness and manipulating reality and others. Being free of all of that because you're embracing a larger reality of love and compassion, kindness. So I think that renunciation is really an initiation into a process of sensitivity, greater and greater sensitivity. It's a letting go of one thing in order to be, develop, cultivate something much, much more expansive and of benefit to all.

TC   It's a renunciation, as I said at the beginning, of suffering. We're also renouncing distractions, so that we will have the mental time and space to turn toward what's meaningful and what's important in life.

SR   For me, I just know that with renunciation my life has expanded and so has my vision. It's a dynamic process of evolving consciousness. When I took *sanyas,* I began to understand that there was a lot more to renunciation than letting things go. It's a commitment to facing life and moving forward.

CM   Not all of us can take vows or dedicate our lives to renunciation. What are some practical ways that everyday people can practise renunciation?

TC   The first thing is to simplify one's lifestyle. Even though renunciation is an inner attitude, it should be displayed in how we live. When we renounce suffering and its causes, when we renounce selfishness, how do we express that in our lifestyle? Living more simply and not consuming more than our fair share of the world's resources. Seeing our impact on the environment and other beings, we become more mindful and reduce our consumption, reuse what we have, and recycle.

SR   On a more subtle level, people can also renounce the images they hold of people who are close to them or people as they meet them, by suspending judgement. This allows people to change and for their fullness to come forward. A lot of times, people are attached to their ideas and concepts, and they are very hard to let go of. But sometimes something will come in to help you in the right direction. Here in BC this summer, with the forest fires, people have had to ask, "What am I going to take with me?" as they were evacuated from their homes. The community has become really strong in helping each other. Things aren't as important. Compassion and caring become the focus.

WT   We can have a very, very committed, disciplined, regular practice. Like meditation. A practice of mindfulness in each moment. I think renunciation is a practice in meeting people. It's just to accept them. You don't accept their actions, but you accept them as a person. By constantly evaluating people, it's a diminishment of the other. So instead of engaging in diminishing the other, you just accept them as like yourself and don't make any judgement about where they're at and just be there, present for them. And you know, if they need something in terms of insight or encouragement or love and acceptance, then they will ask for that. So I think that's a positive way to practise renunciation in human relationships.

CM   All three of you have made commitments to the path of renunciation. When you did that, I want to ask you how your lives changed.

TC I became much clearer. I gained clarity during the process of deciding that I wanted to make a commitment and take Buddhist monastic vows. I had more direction in life and clear ethical discipline. I didn't justify and rationalize my harmful actions and had less distraction from practising the path. So, mentally, it had a big impact on me at the beginning. As I've practised over time, the commitment has transformed into an opportunity to serve, a commitment to carrying these teachings on to future generations.

CM Brother Wayne, what happened in your life?

WT Well, you know, it's still happening! Let me tell you a short little story. When I was a novice many years ago, one of the professors, Father Damon, who was quite a mystic in his own right, was teaching us a course in spirituality. He said to us, "Don't give yourself to God in one great act of self-donation, of youthful idealism, because you'll end up taking yourself back bit by bit. Be sure of what you're surrendering; be sure that you're fully ready in your generosity to let something go." I think transformation is a lifetime's work or perhaps many lifetimes' work. That's one thing.

More and more as I've gone along, I realize I'm not here for me. It's not a question of Brother Wayne as Brother Wayne. By living the commitment, I am helping others in their struggles. The three of us, along with all others who have chosen this monastic life of renunciation, are signs of the ultimate quest. Of the urgency of that ultimate way of life and that everyone has to come to it sooner or later. So, in that sense, we're ambassadors of the spiritual life. By living it, we are evaluated and judged and criticized and praised, all of which is irrelevant, but it's serving a larger social function, in the *sangha,* in the Christian community, in the Hindu community, for the whole world. And furthermore, I feel that renunciation is a way in which I can become more fully available to what the Christian tradition calls *agathic* love, selfless love, not selfish love. So in those ways I've noticed the changes.

CM And Swami Radhananda, how has your life changed?

SR   The initiation into *sanyas* is just a beginning. I'm trying to establish the Light deeply and to be generous with it, with what I've gained from my personal experience and from these teachings. Renunciation is like a signpost for others, because once a commitment is made, other people either turn toward it or against it. It's like the commitment is so strong, they can see it in action, through the teaching and through living it. I feel that I'm just beginning to understand this path. So I'm always thinking and giving from that place of learning. Then I take another step. It's just such a joy that everything I do could be taken as worship. Then I have something to give that's really worthwhile.

CM   *The word "renunciation" is very similar to the words "enunciation" and "pronunciation." It does seem to me as if renouncing is almost like a declaration, an act of speech in some way. Would you agree with that?*

WT   Yes, it is, it's a declaration. I'm more and more struck by how conversion or transformation is such a long process. In a sense, it could be achieved in a second, but the foundation necessary takes time. I have to say that I think in our day and age what we're doing is very necessary because Radhananda and Chodron and I and you live in a culture that is very, very unsupportive of really serious spiritual life. In some sense, it's an uphill struggle and more and more reminders are needed. I'm very conscious that, yes, we serve a public function and we're not in that position for ourselves.

SR   Especially in receiving a spiritual name, it's saying that we're on a different path. And to me it's a constant reminder and support that I have changed and I'm making it public. So the spiritual work can only come out through my actions. The promise in the name that I've been given is that I keep the teachings visible.

TC   Yes, it is a declaration. In one way, it's a declaration to myself, saying to myself that now living in ethical discipline, developing compassion and love, and opening my heart are most important in my life. It's a declaration to others in many ways. For example, I wear robes, I shave my head. It declares to men that if they want to relate to me, they can't do it in a sexual way. So it completely transforms my relationships with the opposite sex.

In addition, monastic life is a symbol of hope in a society that's so torn by war and poverty. Just knowing that there are people trying to transform their hearts and minds, and people who are consciously developing a kind heart and wisdom – just knowing that gives people in this society a sense of hope and inspiration.

CM   So you renounce society's ideas of joys and pleasure; you are a public symbol of spiritual intent. Can I ask then, is it a good life?

TC   Yes, definitely. I'm actually much happier now than I was before. My mind is much more peaceful and much more open, definitely. We're not renouncing happiness; we're cultivating a type of joy that comes from within and doesn't depend on having things, attaining status or position, or being praised. There is an internal sense of well-being and a wish to share that with others.

SR   It's a joy! To be in the company of the wise, to be with people who are also trying to bring the Light into the world; it's so engaging and real.

CM   Brother Wayne, is it a good life?

WT   I think so. I would agree with that; it's a joy, but sometimes it's a tough joy!

TC   Yes!

SR   That's true!

WT   It's not very easy. There is incredible happiness and one knows that this is the way. But there are so many distractions in the culture, and temptations come up and then you kind of go, "Well, am I crazy or something?" It's a tough joy, but I know in the depths of my being, to put it in Christian terms, this is the will of God for me. I've always felt this sense of call. That in the long run we may think we have a choice, but it's truly decided by the reality of the Divine. ॐ

[About the participants:

Bhikshuni Thubten Chodron *spent most of her early life near Los Angeles where she studied and worked as a schoolteacher before devoting her life to Buddhist teachings. Her initial contact with Buddhism inspired her to face the challenges of her daily life. After many years of study, Chodron received full ordination as a nun in l986.*

Having lived and taught in Asia, Europe, Latin America and Israel, Chodron is now based in Washington State establishing Sravasti Abbey. The abbey is a spiritual community where monastics and those preparing for ordination, male and female, can practise according to Tibetan Buddhist tradition. Chodron is a great supporter of monasticism as a path of liberation and selfless service. "There is much joy in ordained life," she explains, "and it comes from looking honestly at our own condition as well as at our potential. We have to commit to going deeper and peeling away the many layers of hypocrisy, clinging and fear inside ourselves. We are challenged to jump into empty space and to live our faith and aspiration."

Swami Radhananda *is a yogini,* ascent *columnist and spiritual director of Yasodhara Ashram in Kootenay Bay, BC. She met her spiritual teacher, Swami Sivananda Radha, in 1977. "At the time," she says, "I was struggling with an underlying feeling of absence in my life. I was married, had two children and a career – but something was still missing." Swami Radha's teachings touched her immediately. "She spoke about the purpose of life and how to live life fully. She spoke about bringing quality and Light into every aspect of our lives."*

For many years Radhananda lived as a householder yogi, integrating the philosophy and practices of yoga into her work as mother, teacher and education consultant. She became president of Yasodhara Ashram in 1993 and was initiated into the order of sanyas *soon after. As a swami, her main concern has been making the teachings of yoga accessible to everyday practitioners, especially youth.*

Today Radhananda devotes her time to writing, teaching and supporting a widespread community of students and teachers in reaching their potential through self-reflection and the study of yoga.

Brother Wayne Teasdale *was a lay monk, author and teacher. In 1986 he responded to a call from his close friend and teacher, Father Bede Griffiths, the English Benedictine monk who pioneered interreligious thought and practice. Brother Wayne*

determined to be free   133

traveled to Griffiths' ashram in India and was initiated as a Christian sanyasi. *Following the initiation he expressed a wish to stay at the ashram, but Griffiths encouraged him to return home. "You're needed in America, not here in India," Griffiths said. "The real challenge for you is to be a monk in the world, a* sanyasi *who lives in the midst of society, at the very heart of things."*

Brother Wayne carried out the counsel of his teacher by pursuing a mystic path while making a living and working for social justice. Brother Wayne passed away in the fall of 2004.]

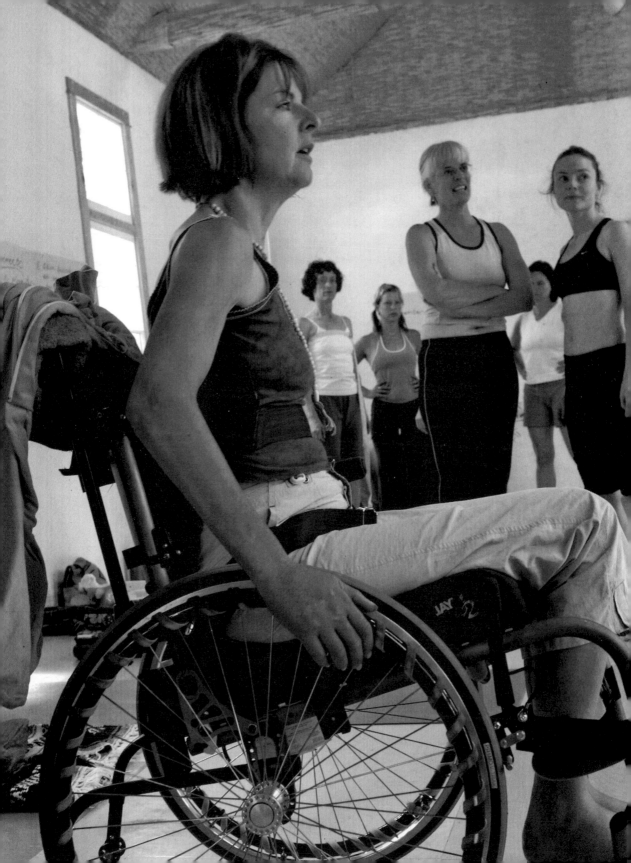

First published in Issue 24, Health & Healing, Winter 2004

mary-jo

how a yogini, & her community, heals: a student's journal

[by Eileen Delehanty Pearkes]

Day 1

I find a place on the floor in a tidy, white-walled yoga studio, with stained-glass windows creating rosy light and a ceiling covered by bamboo mats arching overhead. It is just before 8 a.m. on the first day of a six-day teacher training workshop. My mat and those of the fourteen other participants are arranged like flower petals around the room. The workshop will be led by Jennifer Steed and Mary-Jo Fetterly, the founders of Trinity Yoga.

On Sunday, January 25, 2004, Mary-Jo Fetterly was skiing at Whitewater Mountain in the South Selkirk Range near Nelson, BC. Encouraged by acquaintances to go to "the backside" of the mountain, where untracked powder and steep slopes beckoned, Mary-Jo decided to follow them onto a path, but she caught an edge on its gently undulating surface and flipped through the air. She landed on her head, sustaining severe damage to the C-5, C-6 and C-7 vertebrae.

photo by Rik Logtenberg

A few weeks before her accident, I had spent a Saturday morning with Mary-Jo in this same studio, learning about Manipura Chakra, "City of the Shining Jewel." The third chakra, Mary-Jo taught us, is "the key to the esteemed self," the gateway between the physical and spiritual worlds. I recall her words and the image of her exquisitely strong, flexible body, demonstrating the Scissors pose. Balanced on her two hands, she extended one leg out behind her and brought the other leg forward over its corresponding shoulder. After watching her easily enter the pose and hold it for several breaths, we attempted to do the same. Despite her careful instructions about how to enter and hold the pose, none of us could match her strength and we quickly collapsed into laughter and a tangle of yoga mats.

As we wait quietly for Mary-Jo to arrive, I think about the dramatic changes in her body. She now has no sensation in her abdomen or middle spine, the region associated with the Manipura Chakra. Medical doctors predict that she will never do the Scissors pose again, or even walk, for that matter. She is confined to a wheelchair. She needs support from pillows or straps on her wheelchair even to sit erect. She is as atypical a yoga teacher now as she was once typical, with her mastery of poses, her vibrant teaching style and her enthusiasm for the integration of body, mind and spirit.

Right after the Manipura Chakra workshop in early January, Mary-Jo urged me to take a teacher training course with her. I had studied Ashtanga Yoga with her for four years, had a steady home practice and moved with a certain amount of confidence and poise, even if I had not mastered some of the more challenging poses in the primary series of the Ashtanga system. Why did her suggestion surprise me? Why did I feel hesitant? Perhaps an understanding that I needed a great deal of formal training to be a responsible yoga teacher, and that I didn't have room in my life for what that would require. Perhaps a view of myself as not being capable. *I'm offering a teacher training in Nelson in the spring,* Mary-Jo had said, contradicting my internal doubts. *You should take it. You are ready.*

Then, a few weeks after our conversation, the accident happened. A teacher training workshop with her seemed less than a remote possibility. *Don't you study with Mary-Jo Fetterly?* a friend asked me the day after the accident. *She's fallen, and she's been air-ambulanced to Vancouver General's spinal cord unit.* I can recall pressing the phone harder into my ear, as if to hear something different, rather than the shocking truth. Mary-Jo? How could she, of all people, fall? *It's not possible,* I said.

But it was. The woman who had served as a powerful mental, physical and spiritual model for me and many others had fallen. She was very near death. News of the tragedy flew around our tight-knit community. Then, in the immediate and longer aftermath of an event no one could have predicted, the meaning of yoga began to expand.

I hear a rustle behind me at the studio entrance. Mary-Jo's daughter and a close friend carry her in on a sling created by their arms. They lower her onto a gel cushion and begin to arrange pillows behind her. I measure the muscular power and grace she once possessed against this, her small and vulnerable form being settled into a seated position. Of course, I know that yoga is not just about the body, that the source of this woman's inspiration is not and never has been physical. Yet tears well in my eyes. My heart thumps uncomfortably against the reality of her condition. She appears as a shadow of her former self.

Day 2

The next morning, seated in her wheelchair, Mary-Jo speaks to us of the accident. Her grace rises through her words. Her eyes are clear and shining, her chest open to the world, her voice soft but strong. She looks healthy and she speaks with clarity, despite all that she has been through in the past several months: major spinal surgery, a respirator, hours and hours of challenging therapy and rehabilitation.

"Consciousness," she says, "holds a space that transcends physical reality."

"I have learned a new appreciation of the physical form, of the human ability to feel," she adds. Her partially paralyzed hands lift off the wheels of the chair in a stiff but expressive swirl. "My yoga practice, from the moment I fell until now, has been a source of strength and a guide. It kept me alive as I lay in the snow feeling the paralysis take hold and realized I must rely on breathing from the diaphragm in order to live. It enabled me to move out of the spinal cord unit in half the usual time," she says. Then she pauses and looks around the room. Using her arms to brace herself, she leans slightly forward in her chair. "I have come to realize that we are doing so little with our freedom and our capacity."

Later, as she leads us through a series of *asanas,* I am surrounded as if wrapped in a comforting blanket by her words. In a culture that relentlessly pursues the physical aspects of yoga, sometimes with the goal to create the "perfect body," that body can so easily become a trap, rather than a springboard to freedom.

I realize as I move through numerous Sun Salutations, then Triangle, Side Angle and Half-Moon, that I cannot really sense Mary-Jo's physical presence in the room. She is there, in her wheelchair. I am here, and others surround me, but I must make an effort to hold on to this perception. Her intuitive grasp of the body and its alignment remains identical in her teaching. I realize, though, that the absence of her form demonstrating poses or striding through the mats to energize the room has had an effect. From the limitation of her wheelchair, she seems to be capable of leading us to a limitless place, beyond the room, beyond the mats and the limbs we control.

During a lunch break, I puzzle over the wonderful feeling the *asana* series has left me with. I have felt something inexplicable, something like the Divine. I ask other workshop participants about it. One describes Mary-Jo's teaching as having become "completely whole." Her comment makes intuitive sense to me, but also suggests an irony that I puzzle over further. How could Mary-Jo's teaching be whole, if she herself is no longer WHOLE. If she is, in the words of our culture, "disabled"?

Later that night, I ease my stiff body into a bath of Epsom salts, thinking again about wholeness and yoga. The news of Mary-Jo's accident initially shattered the yoga community in and around Nelson. Tragedy does this. Yet, once the truth had been absorbed and the shards of grief and loss were scattered chaotically about, an opportunity arose to draw together. The willingness to pick up the pieces and create a new whole exposed our community to a sort of yoga few had experienced, a yoga that was fresh, though ancient, a yoga alive with possibility.

A few days after the accident, a close friend of Mary-Jo's called a prayer circle. Forty people gathered in the town's largest yoga studio, a studio Mary-Jo had helped create several years earlier. There, in the dark of a winter night, healing thoughts and prayer created a flame around which we could cup our collective hands.

By the end of the first week after the accident, Mary-Jo had been removed from the respirator. She had survived long, complex surgeries to stabilize her spine. An avalanche of cards, flowers, letters and gifts began to arrive at the Vancouver hospital where she lay. Emails came in by the dozens. She was alive, and she was improving, by the smallest amount. Her website became an information pipeline for updated news of her condition, with eloquent web logs posted frequently by her eldest daughter Amanda. Her students and others, even people who had never taken a yoga class, checked the website regularly.

The room where I practise yoga did not have an altar before Mary-Jo's accident. I had toyed for a few years with creating one, but had never gotten around to it. In the worrisome days of late winter, my small studio seemed incomplete without one. I rummaged in a box from a recent move. I found a ceramic statue of Kuanyin, Chinese goddess of compassion. I placed her on the windowsill and in front of her set a small votive candle.

With self-consciousness swept aside by concern for another, I lit a candle at the start of my practice each day. Guided by the peaceful face of Kuanyin, I offered soft breath and compassion to Mary-Jo's suffering as I moved my own healthy body through the *asana* series she had taught me. In these efforts, the Divine entered my practice. Something beyond the grasp of any of us had arrived to help us pick up the shards of grief and yoke them together, to bring meaning to the loss.

Day 3

I wake to sore muscles and a scattered mind. My stomach aches and I am tired. I would like to stay in bed, but I rise to get breakfast organized for my family before heading off to more lectures and demonstrations. Today, as a group, we will design a ninety-minute class for the general public. I suspect that this exercise will lead to us teaching that same class to the public later in the week. I feel unenthusiastic about both possibilities. My uncertainties about being "ready" to train as a yoga teacher are being exposed.

In *The Heart of Yoga*, Desikachar discusses "the nine obstacles on the yoga way." These are *antarayas*, or rocks, lying on the path, impositions to progress. They are listed by Patanjali in the Yoga Sutras: illness, lethargy, doubt, haste or impatience, resignation or fatigue, distraction, ignorance or arrogance, inability to take a new step, and loss of confidence.

The eighth of these, *alabdhabhumikatva,* the inability to take a new step, had begun to plague me. Just as one feels one has made some progress, a voice of doubt arises, suggesting that there is still so much to learn or do that it could not be a step one is capable of taking. This, along with the ninth obstacle, *anavasthitatvani,* or lack of confidence, pulled at my focus as I sat perched on a folded blanket during morning meditation. What was I doing here? How could I possibly stand in front of a class to teach when I felt that I still knew so little?

Before we take on the task of designing a class, Mary-Jo speaks to us briefly from her nest of pillows on the floor. "When something changes physically, there is a cultural assumption that one loses capability." The references to her condition are obvious. But like any good teacher, Mary-Jo continues, summarizing the best approach to any rock one might find in one's path, regardless of age, ability or health. "Don't let your mind or conceptions hold you back in your life from giving what you are meant to offer."

I think of wheelchair ramps, urine bags and the struggle to accomplish even the simplest of life tasks independently. To hear these words from Mary-Jo reminds me that my own doubts are simply conceptions, not truths. If she can be here, teaching a course a mere six months after her accident, what can I be doing that I have not allowed myself to achieve? I settle in with the rest of the group to discuss posture sequencing. When it comes time to divide the poses among us and I am arbitrarily given two poses to teach that are not my strongest, I accept them with as much grace as I can muster.

The ability of yoga to remove obstacles found its full expression in our community in the months following Mary-Jo's accident. A single mother of two daughters, Mary-Jo depended on the income her teaching generated. As the extreme nature of her injuries became apparent, worries arose about how she would support and educate her teenage daughters, about what the future would hold for them.

Members of the community stepped forward to organize a silent auction fundraiser to take place at the end of February, to contribute to a trust fund established to ameliorate losses. One by one, the typical obstacles for running a successful fundraiser rolled aside like small pebbles. Donations to the silent auction poured in with little promotional effort. As the number of donations outgrew the location, a local hotel stepped in to offer its largest banquet room free of charge.

The night of the event, hundreds milled around the room and by the end of the evening, $27,500 had been raised. Even those who did not know Mary-Jo very well or practise much yoga spoke with amazement about the love and positive spirit in the room. Where had it come from, they wondered?

The heart of yoga spread throughout the community in a way that could not have been anticipated. The willingness to give, and then give more, and then more again, was a sign of hearts opening, more than could be counted. Mary-Jo, who had touched dozens of people through her work as a yoga teacher, was suddenly touching more through her accident. In return, she and her family were being supported and comforted by the generosity of many. The event and its enormous success attracted the attention of national media. *What kind of community is it that unites to help out so quickly in such a significant way?* one reporter asked. *I think I'd like to live there.*

Day 4

We focus on restorative yoga. We practise it for over an hour, with piles of pillows, bolsters and blankets to use as support systems in several deeply relaxing, supine poses. At the end, we settle in to *Savasana*, which seems redundant after all the other restorative poses. I am surprised to find myself an adept corpse. When the chimes ring and I am stirred back to life, I realize how hungry for deep surrender my physical body and my mind have been.

Later, I approach Mary-Jo during a break to chat. As she tries to adjust herself in her nest of pillows, she loses her balance and flops forward, into a deep *Pascimottanasana* facilitated by her paralysis. When I comment teasingly on her ability to "surrender into the pose," she lifts her face from the floor and laughs. "Oh, I've surrendered now, baby," she says. "You better believe it."

As spring took hold, the swelling of Mary-Jo's spine following the injury and surgery had reduced to the point that a fairly accurate portrait of the damage could be drawn. It was clear that despite her remarkable health and well-being prior to the accident, Mary-Jo's ability to recover from the spinal damage would, for now at least, be limited by the physical realities of her broken vertebrae and the damaged nerves. She had good function from the chest up, with excellent shoulder and elbow mobility, a small amount of finger dexterity and a faint sensation in her left foot. She could feed herself, with a spoon or fork strapped to her wrist.

Yet rumours in the community about her "miraculous recovery" persisted, including one that she was walking again. The rumours seemed to fuel a desire to hold on to the image of Mary-Jo that we had become attached to, that of an athletic woman who could inspire us and lead us as we had grown accustomed.

About that time, a few people organized another, smaller fundraiser for the trust fund, an evening of mantra singing and a talk about a spiritual community in India. Sixty people gathered, some of whom had never chanted a mantra before. Voices swelled and filled the darkened room. Minds grew quiet. Collectively, we contemplated the possibility that Mary-Jo might be transforming in a way that required us, as well as her, to surrender.

Day 5

We perform a dry run of our first yoga class, each of us taking a few of the poses. We are nervous and uncertain about our offerings. When my turn comes, I step up to teach *Navasana* (the Boat) and Table pose, two *asanas* I might have viewed as nearly impossible to do, let alone teach, as little as two years ago. It is not an accident that I have been given these two poses to teach, I realize, but a message from the Divine.

I speak to the imaginary class about how core strength creates its own lifeboat, allowing us to handle the unpredictable and wavelike nature of the mind, and of life. Sitting on the mat at the front of the room, I realize for the first time the full significance of the boat, of weathering stormy seas through balance and strength from the core of one's body and being.

Afterward, I think of Mary-Jo. How is it that she has been able to weather the seas she has traveled in the past several months, to be strong enough to surrender to the divinity of her injury? Before the accident, she could hold *Navasana* for long stretches, while giving us inspiration to hold our own boats steady. Now, though she is paralyzed, her core strength continues to see her through. She draws brilliant Light from the Manipura Chakra and sends its sparkling nature into the world.

Day 6

How do I step gracefully across the divide between student and teacher? Perhaps in the same way that Mary-Jo has surrendered so graciously to her new physical limitations, with faith and trust in the Divine.

Preparing over the past week to teach a portion of the public class – my first small and nerve-wracking teaching experience – turns out to be a process of self-revelation as much as an opportunity to develop what Desikachar calls *asmita*, the ego's voice that says, "I am a yoga teacher."

What does that voice really mean? The seventy hours of instruction have been an important beginning. They have taught me that becoming a teacher is as much about accessing an empowered inner being as it is about the technicalities of yoga, with its alignments, muscle groups and posture sequences.

In this, Mary-Jo has been a superb example and guide. How to practise yoga, from a wheelchair, on a mat, touching one's toes – or not – in a traffic jam, at the park, as a mother, as a grocery clerk, during an argument, after an illness, or sometimes, as the wail of a tragedy echoes around a mountain valley, calling people awake, reminding them of truth, introducing them again to the heart of human experience.

Coda: Patanjali, Sutra 1.7

In a state of yoga, comprehension is different from comprehension at other times. It is closer to the true nature of the object. ॐ

[UPDATE: Mary-Jo Fetterly now lives in Vancouver with her two daughters, where she guides the development of Trinity Yoga. She now sits on the advisory panel for the Rick Hansen Spinal Cord Registry, an international information centre for research and development into quality of life for those who have spinal cord injury.]

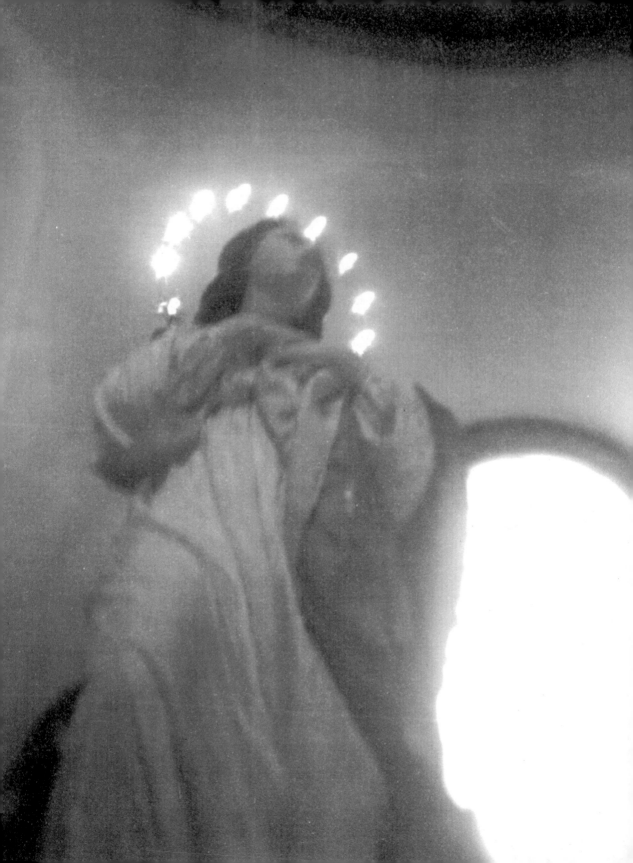

First published in Issue 10, Bhakti, Summer 2001

butter tart bliss

being on anne brothers' prayer list

[by Clea McDougall]

for about three weeks now, I've been on Anne's prayer list. Each night, around eleven o'clock, the image of an eighty-year-old woman kneeling down next to her bed for her nightly prayers sneaks into my mind. I don't yet know how to tell if her prayers are working, but almost beyond my will I check myself out each day, looking for a change, a new sense of peace, something.

My own Catholic inheritance ended when the Roman Catholic church refused to let my Italian grandmother get married in the "House of God" because she was already pregnant at the time. She was so mad that she swore off Catholicism for the rest of her life. I think something of this spirit still lingers in my blood, and I've never felt connected to Catholicism. I have been studying yoga for many years now and see prayer in a contemplative way. I pray or meditate or practise yoga to understand myself and to control my mind. It's an abstract understanding, but it seems it suits me and my mind.

Anne, on the other hand, is much more concrete in her devotion. She prays

photo by Clea McDougall

to certain saints or holy figures *for* certain things. She prays for the well-being of others. She prays for her family, her close friends, the priests she looks after, and anyone who tells her they are in need of her prayers. When I asked her why she does this, she answered simply, "Well, now, because I enjoy it."

Anne Brothers is the live-in housekeeper and cook at the Holy Cross Parish rectory in Kemptville, Ontario. She is well known around town for her prayers and her famous butter tarts, which are some of the sweetest and butteriest and most delicious tarts you will ever taste. Her generosity with both her prayers and her tarts inspires some people to call her Saint Anne. She also happens to be the grandmother of a good friend of mine and that is how I got the chance to meet her.

Sarah and I arrived in Kemptville at eleven o'clock one Sunday morning in late spring. The Salvation Army store greeted us with a big JESUS LOVES YOU sign as we drove up the main strip. There was no one on the streets, but a church on almost every corner, and I suspected the townspeople to be all snuggled inside them for various Sunday services.

The rectory is a large stone house beside an even larger stone church. A white stone Jesus with open arms stands in the middle of the church grounds, and faces out toward the small valley town. I was a little nervous about this whole trip, spending a day with priests and praying grandmothers, but Sarah reassured me that I would be fine, and so I followed her into the rectory. There was Anne, standing down the hall, framed by her bright kitchen, calling to us in her heavy English lilt, "Where have you been, Sarah? I've been expecting you, my pet. Don't bother taking your shoes off, the floor's a wee bit cold."

She looks like any regular grandmother. You can see the shadow of her granddaughter, Sarah, in her face, although the top of her head comes to below Sarah's shoulder, and she has that great thinning hair all women of eighty seem to have. A Tupperware mountain full of butter tarts, muffins and scones sat on the counter. After she welcomed us in with a hug and a kiss, Anne indicated that these were for Sarah to take back with her. "Yesterday I made three dozen muffins, three dozen scones and five dozen tarts. So these are for you." She turned to me and added, "And I packed a little box of butter tarts for you dear, just your own."

Anne makes about 200 tarts each week. Her secret recipe has been in the making for twenty-two years. She distributes them throughout the town to people who, for some reason or another, have found themselves on Anne's butter tart list, including the inmates at the local prison. Anne also ships the tarts in care packages around the world. Her tarts have been called the physical manifestation of her prayer life. There *is* something almost magical about them, you can't help feeling she's made them just for you.

As Sarah and I sat and drank tea, Anne clanked around us. Her kitchen felt like the centre of the world. The neighbouring Holy Cross Church filled all the windows, and you could almost feel the quiet of Sunday mass pushing into the kitchen. Absolutely nothing stirred in this town but Anne, dishes clanking, soup burning, lunch being prepared. She chatted to us all the while, reciting her eightieth birthday speech, showing us her rosaries, making us toast and giggling as she pulled out her secret stash of Guinness. We tried to get her to sit down with us, but she wouldn't hear of it. I asked her if she ever stops working, but she didn't answer me.

Anne Donnelly Brothers was born in 1920, in Durham county, England, to Irish immigrant parents. She was the fourth of nine children, part of a large Catholic family. When she was ten years old, she had a vivid experience of seeing Mary. She and her baby brother Michael contracted pneumonia at the same time. "I was lyin' in bed – we were both in the same room – Michael was in the cot, I was in the bed and John, me other brother who was six at the time, he's dead now, he was sitting by my bed. I said to him, 'Oh, look, John, there's Our Blessed Lady!' Mary was on the wall, you see. I said, 'I must be going to die.' He jumped up and ran out of the room. Mary stood there for a few seconds. She was dressed in a very, very shell-pink dress, with a blue cloak and a white veil. She had dark hair. I'm not sure the colour of her eyes, but she was beautiful." Anne recalled this in a cooing voice, still full of awe, lost in the memory. "Mary disappeared and a few minutes later she came back, at the foot of my bed, and she was lookin' at me. She never spoke, she never moved, she was so beautiful, and then she disappeared. I got better and Michael died. The Blessed Virgin came for him, you see."

"I'll always remember that," she continues. "I can often see her. When I'm prayin', I can see her in me mind's eye, just as she was. Oooo, she was very beautiful."

During the Second World War, she joined the air force as a general duty officer. She taught dance classes to the airmen and it was in the air force that she met her future husband, Mike Brothers. They were married in 1943 and lived in a house five doors down from where she grew up, and where her parents still lived.

Mike and Anne had one child, a daughter. The family moved to Canada in October of 1953, sailing over on the maiden voyage of the *Olympia,* docking in New York and driving up to Toronto where they lived for five years. They then moved to Trenton, Ontario, where Mike started up a local road-oiling business and built a house on the outskirts of town. Mike Brothers died in 1973. The business was too much for Anne to manage by herself, so she sold it and the house and moved into an apartment in downtown Trenton.

At age fifty-six, when most people think about retiring, Anne started a new career.

"In 1976, Father Lynette came to the apartment and asked me to be his housekeeper. He had fired the other housekeeper, because she was always fightin' with him, but that made his stomach bad, you know, he's very humble. This was in December, and I go home to see my daughter and her family every Christmas. So I agreed to come back on the second of January.

"On that morning, he was sayin' mass, so I went to mass and waited for him, and we walked over to the rectory together and I've been with him ever since. I've been with him twenty-four years now. I moved with him from Trenton here to Kemptville. I work six days a week lookin' after Father Lynette and Father Augustane. And it's been a wonderful life, I've enjoyed every day and the more there is to attend to the better. Yes, it's a great life, I thank God for it."

"She's a Pray-er. That's just what she is," Sarah explains. "When I was a child, I used to think my grandmother was crazy. There would always be this murmur murmur murmur coming from her. I thought she was just talking to herself. It used to scare me. It wasn't until I was much older that I found out she was praying. She prays all day long."

And Anne's prayers are often sought after. Even Father Lynette brings people through into the kitchen to meet Anne and be put on her prayer list. She recounted a story in which she prayed for one of her favourite priests as he was driving home during a snowstorm. He hit a patch of ice, spun around four times and realized he was facing the traffic head on, but luckily was on the shoulder of the road. The next morning at mass, he told the whole congregation to never underestimate the power of prayer, and that Anne Brothers' prayers were powerful.

"I have a list about this long," Anne measured about the length of her forearm. "I pray in the morning, I have a bunch of prayers there that I read every morning. I pray me rosary during the day, and I read prayers, and every now and again during the day I ask the Lord to guide everybody, to keep them safe, grant them the grace to do well and be successful.

"I pray for Sarah, always, to keep her safe from danger or accidents and guide her away from drinking, drugs or bad influences. But some people ask for very, very special intentions, now for instance, to sell a house. People asked me a couple of months ago to pray for them to sell the house. Well, I did, and it sold. Then I prayed that they'd get a nice house. And they did. So that was prayers answered."

I wanted an explanation, but Anne knocks down my questions with simple answers. Me: Have you always had faith? Anne: Oh yes, I've been a Catholic all my life. Me: So you can pray for anything? Anne: Oh yes, anything. I'll pray for you from now on, dear. Me: And if the prayers don't work? Anne: Well, it wasn't God's will.

An admirer of Christian meditation, Father Lynette is a kind and open-minded Catholic priest. He likes to golf and told me that a guy by the name of Saint Anthony is a good friend of his, because he always finds his lost golf balls. "I don't pray the same way as Anne does. I use my own words, you know? I see Mary as sort of a spiritual mother. I say, Okay. Hi Mary, Holy Mary, Mother of Jesus. I'm not devout or anything, but I like to talk to Mary." He sees his devotion as more of a commitment – to God and to the Church.

For Father Lynette, prayer itself hasn't made a drastic change in his life, but by listening to the silence of prayer he has come to know his God in a kinder and more personal way. I asked him why he refers his parishioners to Anne for prayers. "We believe that God is spirit, the holy spirit, the spirit of love. Because of Anne's goodwill, she becomes a channel for it."

Sarah has another angle on it. "She's eighty years old, and has been praying all her life. You may start with prayer or whatever to calm your mind or for comfort, but it's like anything, it's got to evolve. I think it's probably evolved for her, how spiritual paths evolve for everyone. She's lived her life, raised a family, and now she can be giving. She lives her prayers every day, she doesn't just go to church once a week. Catholicism is alive for her."

To me, it seems that Anne's prayers have become rooted so deeply in her heart that there is no room for doubt. They are as natural to her as breathing. I've never met a person with such simple and unshakeable faith. My own mind is constantly plagued by questions, everything from the existence of a Divine power to my own relation to it. But Anne accepts what is. She finds so much joy in something as simple as saying her rosary, her eyes moisten looking at her favourite picture of Mary. She is simple in her beliefs, but not a simplistic person. By simply believing, she has opened up her life, left room in her mind for happiness.

"Faith is a gift," explains Father Lynette. "Any person who has faith has been given a gift from God." I liked Father Lynette, and I think he heard my silent retort, *But what if you haven't been given the gift of faith?* He continued on, "I believe the fact that you are studying and trying to develop your appreciation of yoga is also a gift. That condition of faith and that desire are gifts."

"See!" Anne pointed to a crucifix on the wall and giggled conspiratorially. Jesus' feet, which should have been in gold leaf like the rest of him, were a worn brown. "I kiss His feet every morning! I've rubbed all the paint off!"

We ended the day sitting in Anne's room and talking about her life. She gave us both a bottle of St. Joseph's oil, saying that it would cure any cut or bruise or ache if you rub it on, or take a bath in it. "Oh, it just feels so good," she promised. Sarah tried to refuse (she has a cabinet full of these gifts already) but Anne wouldn't take no for an answer. Saint Joseph is her favourite saint, and she orders this oil, from Saint Joseph's Cathedral in Montréal, by the caseload. She's a bit on the eccentric side, but so are most women of eighty years. She's allowed to be. She started rifling off her prayers again for us.

"I say the Hail Holy Queen, and Praise Our Blessed Lady. And I always say Jesus, guide our family and our children from danger and accidents and keep them safe, wherever they may be.

"Now, at night, I have an Our Lady, Our Redeemer prayer – she helps you. I pray to Saint Jude, Saint Peregrine, as I said, for cancer patients, Saint Teresa the little flower, Our Lady of Sorrows, Father Fredrick, he's for alcoholics and drug dependencies. I say the Legion of Mary prayers, as I told you, and me rosary, and then I kneel on me knees for about an hour and twenty minutes, sometimes more, all depends on how many I've got to pray for, and I usually get to bed about twelve o'clock. I think it was five to twelve last night when I went to bed. Of course, I take a bath in the meantime, phone me family and friends and from seven o'clock, when I finish me work, to twelve o'clock, time flies."

She pauses and looks thoughtful. "I guess that's me story."

I left the Holy Cross Parish that day with more questions than I arrived with. There is a part of me that is skeptical and a part that is distrustful about the Church, but I couldn't help clutching my little Tetley tea box full of butter tarts on the way home. There is something in me that wants to believe, maybe not in the Catholic God, but in the power of prayer. The biggest question that kept repeating itself, in response to Father Lynette, was what if I haven't been given the gift of faith? Sure, I have the desire to study, but how far does that go without faith?

What will happen now that I'm on Anne's prayer list? Despite my doubts, I feel that *something* will happen. There is one point in our visit that still stands out vividly in my mind. We are sitting in her room, and Anne is listing, again, all the saints she prays to, and she is talking to Sarah about family and people I don't know. I just watch Anne. I get a little lost in her pooly old eyes. She is at peace with simplicity; she can love without question. For a slight moment, I am not in the room at all, the world opens up and I see Anne at all the different stages of her life – a girl, a young woman, a mother, an ancient woman – and I understand how much her mind holds and why. On the outside she is a grandmother like any other, but she gave me a glimpse of something else, of a life steeped in prayer. ॐ

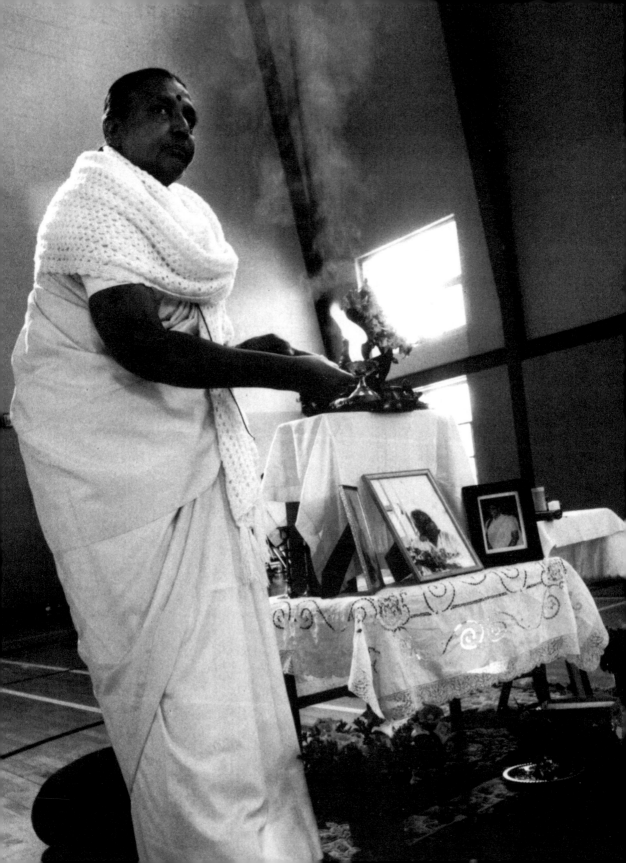

First published in Issue 12, Science, Winter 2001

fire works

an elemental investigation sparked by geeta iyengar

[by Juniper Glass]

i am standing in a Hatha Yoga pose called Warrior. My knees and hips burn. I think, this is enough. I am trying my hardest but I can't see how holding the pose for so long could be good for me.

The teacher, Dr. Geeta Iyengar, has told us that in *asana* practice the mind is stilled because all thoughts gravitate to the body. My mind is consumed by the experience my body is going through. Far from being calm, however, I feel as though I am clamouring just to stay above water.

One of the teacher's assistants steps behind me. My front knee is shaking, but he indicates for me to bend it further. What? I think. I've gone as far as I can. The joints in my legs are prone to injury and I am doing my best to protect them.

Subtly and strongly, another thought enters my mind. It is of a very different nature than the habitual nervous caution, something like – If I'm going to do this, I'm going to do it. I stop listening to the anxious thought that says my knees are too sensitive for the pose. Instead, I listen to my knees.

photo by Nancy Bleck & Susan Stewart

As the bend in my leg deepens, the *asana* becomes much more comfortable. I have a strong body! My torso, limbs and head shift and suddenly feel at home. In the Warrior pose, I sense my body anew. Happiness rushes through me at this discovery: my body is finding a place of its own.

Fire starts with an infusion of energy.
A spark is needed.
Once initiated fire is self-sustaining.

"Conference" conjures an image of stiff surroundings and lots of talk, but this event was meant for experiencing yoga, not just discussing it. During each of the five days of the National Iyengar conference, 300 or so participants filled a gymnasium to practise *pranayama* and *asana* as a group. Dr. Iyengar herself taught most of the classes, which were lengthy and rigorous. Geetaji, as her students call her, was making her first visit to Canada. Energy was certainly high.

I have practised yoga for five years, but this was my first encounter with the Iyengar method. To counter the trepidation I felt at being a newcomer, I reminded myself determinedly that I would find something that I could use in my life. I knew I was lucky for the opportunity to learn from a woman for whom yoga has been a way of life since childhood.

Geeta Iyengar, who I could easily describe as a ball of fire, encourages her students to reach beyond their comfort zone. She would not let anyone give in to weakness. I think she could see the capacity and intelligence concealed within each of us, and she was devoted to helping us find it. Her understanding seemed to be based on a great deal of personal experience.

At age ten, when she had already suffered many childhood illnesses, Geeta became seriously sick again. When she came home from the hospital, her father refused to buy the long list of medications that doctors had prescribed. He told her she would have to choose between the illness, which might mean her death, and yoga practice.

Geetaji faced a great challenge at a young age and found the power within to survive and thrive. She has since devoted her entire life to yoga, becoming one of the foremost teachers of the Iyengar Method of Yoga, which was founded by her father, B.K.S. Iyengar.

Although Geetaji's story is very different from my own, it inspired me to make a stretch. Could it be that things I perceive as hard and fast realities – like how far my knee can bend or how little money I have – are, at least in part, a reflection of my mind?

Dr. Iyengar's opening talk immediately caught my attention. She said that we are "missing the gold" if we do *asanas* as a physical practice only. "More than the body, it is the mind which is getting cultured ... Even five minutes in *Savasana* gives a feeling of quietness. If that experience is stored, understood and opened at the right time, we will know how tranquility is brought about."

"The experience," she explained enticingly, "leaves an imprint."

> *Fire results*
> *from the very rapid combination*
> *of fuel and atmospheric oxygen.*
> *Combustion occurs at the*
> *interface*
> *between fuel and flame.*
> *Fire*
> *is an exchange.*

I am lying on my back listening to Geetaji's voice. She is teaching us *pranayama* and wants us to start with the basics. We are in *Savasana*, the Corpse pose, so that our bodies will relax as we focus on the breath.

I can't relax at all. The gymnasium is very cold and lying down in it is even colder. All morning, the gym has been pumped full of cool air by an air-conditioning system that is out of sync with the weather. My impulse is to curl up tight in my blankets.

Geetaji is not disturbed. As much as I wish her to, she does not ask us to get up. Instead, she teaches us to breathe in a way that will generate heat from within, while remaining in the place where we are. She addresses the temperature directly, saying it is just one challenge among many that we face in life.

When Geetaji lays out the options – shrink up, leave the room, or face the cold and do something about it – I realize that the time to start practising is now. I breathe slowly and smoothly. Each inhalation lifts and expands my chest a little more. My mind is no longer occupied by the struggle to keep warm, but soon warmth radiates from the core of my body out to the tips.

"Earth, water, fire, air, ether," Geetaji says another day during *asana* class. "The elements are there in the body."

As we move through a series of poses, Geetaji brings our attention to the regions and sensations in the body associated with each element. I learn that "fire" is what seems to give the lift to my body. As I expand my chest upward, there really does seem to be a fire inside. When this part of my body does its job, keeping me upright and tall, the parts that usually overwork can relax.

I am fascinated by the effortlessness I experience throughout my body when I put in the effort to lift my chest.

> *Fire is an exergonic chemical reaction:*
> *much energy is released.*

I left the Iyengar conference feeling elated. For days, I was relaxed and standing tall. At the time, I was struggling to make my way in a new city, I didn't yet have a job, and my goal of living in an apartment of my own seemed a long way off. But I took home plenty of enthusiasm to face the challenges.

I wondered why I felt so good. It made sense that by putting a lot of energy out, in the form of concentration and physical exertion, I would get a lot back. But that didn't explain the confidence I felt, nor how the spiritual practices had helped bring it about.

If what Geetaji said was true – that positive experiences from yoga practice can be stored as "wealth" in our minds – then I wanted to understand this experience and build on it.

Fire contained a clue. I had a feeling that if I learned more about this element, then I would better understand my experience. Understanding how joy and confidence arose in my mind during yogic practices, Geetaji promised, would increase my capacity to be joyful and confident. I certainly could use more of these qualities in my life.

What is fire? I began to wonder. How does it work in nature? If this element was a wise person, what kind of wisdom would it possess?

When something burns, its atoms must be forced apart.
In liquids, the expansion process
is evaporative boiling
and in solids it is pyrolysis.
Under the influence of fire
states transform.

Tapas is a practice mentioned in many of the prominent old yogic texts, including the Yoga Sutras of Patanjali. The Sanskrit word means "heat." Often translated as "austerity," *tapas* involves intense, focused effort to achieve a spiritual goal.

One of my teachers explained that *tapas* "clears away the dross" from our minds and acts like a magnifying glass in the sun – bringing a great deal of energy to a single point. The power generated can help us break habits or overcome obstacles within.

The Bhagavad Gita states that *tapas* can be practised in relation to the body, mind and speech. Serenity, silence and honesty of purpose are examples of austerities of the mind given in the Gita (XVII, 16).

Sri Aurobindo describes a fiery spiritual force that we can light in our hearts and all other parts of our being. In his *Letters on Yoga*, Aurobindo writes that "*agni* is at once a fire of aspiration, a fire of purification, a fire of *Tapasya*, a fire of transformation. . . *Agni* opens the earth, the physical consciousness, to the Divine Light."

In the Kundalini system, the symbol for the third level of consciousness contains a Fire Wheel. Swami Radha's book, *Kundalini Yoga for the West*, explains that the third chakra is related to emotions, mind, energy, dreams and the sense of sight. This level of consciousness is also closely linked with the power of imagination.

I get the sense that fire is a mover and shaker in the element world. When the yogic texts talk about fire, it comes across as a dynamic force in the mind with great potential to transform.

I get all fired up reading the words of these masters. They make spiritual life sound like alchemy.

Convection currents create
the shape of flames.
On Earth
in an open environment
fresh air is channeled upward
(hot air rises)
resulting in flames that lift.
Moving air makes flames dance.

This weekend, I am moving into a place of my own. It is a basement suite with many quirks like saloon doors and no sink in the bathroom. It is also bright, sun-coloured and mine.

Moving into my own apartment reflects a change happening inside me. I am finding out what it is I seek and mustering up the courage to let it become reality. In order to take steps toward what I want deep down, I have to act outside of habitual ways.

After the conference, I used the enthusiasm I had gained to question myself persistently: What do I seek? What do I want my life to look like? Clarifying the answers was like burning away the chaff to get at what was valuable. I saw that living on my own was important. I knew it would help me, as a young woman, to take responsibility for myself and to find out how I want to live my life.

At the time, I could not see how I would be able to afford an apartment. It took courage simply to accept that, yes, it is possible. The crucial step seemed just to take a mental risk, to be willing to go beyond what was known and comfortable.

Once I knew I wanted my own place, I had to work to find it. Having been told that Vancouver was in a housing crunch, I checked the classified ads almost obsessively for weeks. One day, I was scrambling around town trying to land an apartment, and I stopped for coffee in the neighbourhood where I wanted to live. I noticed just how anxious and tense I had become.

In the process of trying to expand my horizons, I had squeezed my mind tight. I recognized this pattern from my job search. When I finally did get permanent work, it came in a gentle, roundabout way that took effort on my part, but not an anxious struggle.

So I decided to try a new tack, handwriting signs for the community bulletin boards: "SEEKING a 1-bedroom suite in Mount Pleasant." I relaxed. In a few days, after I had almost forgotten about the signs, I got the call from my landlady-to-be.

There is a wonderful momentum gaining as I find out that I am capable of more than I thought. I have come to think of this force as the fire in my life.

When I was struggling in the Warrior pose, I didn't really know why I was there or what I was seeking. But the knowledge was right below the surface. As soon as I challenged myself – the thought was like a spark – the innate strength in my body emerged. Instead of seeing myself as a victim of circumstances, I was participating actively in my life.

To me, fire is a symbol for the power I use to clarify what I want and go after it. It was a step for me just to get out and look for an apartment, but I don't want to live my life trying to force everything. The fiery strength I am discovering is too precious to be wasted on strain, which often doesn't amount to much.

The amount of heat produced in a fire
depends upon the quality of fuel
and how much air is allowed in.
The speed at which a fire can travel depends on the materials available to it.

Since the classes with Geetaji, I have wondered: What is the line between straining and giving myself a healthy shove in the right direction?

The burning sensation in my hips and knees during the first *asana* classes is certainly not the flame I want to stoke in my life. I had pushed myself for unhealthy reasons – to prove myself and because I was worried about not doing the poses rght.

Geetaji challenged us on this level as well. "Why are you here?" she asked. "Do not do the *asana* for me – do it for yourself!"

I was getting in touch with my desire to know, for myself, what I am capable of. Geetaji called this "essential intelligence," the knowing from within.

I am living by myself now because I want to expand and explore. Each risk taken brings more confidence. My desire to grow is like a gentle, slow-burning fire. It is becoming a force of its own.

As electrons cool
in atoms that have become hot by fire
light radiates.

As weather on the West Coast shifts from damp to damper, I am cozy in my new place. The heating system is another strange and endearing feature of the apartment. The awkward, natural gas–fueled appliance is mounted halfway up the living room wall. I like the brand name, Valor, and it produces a lovely, permeating warmth.

"Turn it on or off as you wish," my landlady said when she was first showing me the apartment. "You control the heat."

In coal fires
and the sun
the hottest flames
glow white. ॐ

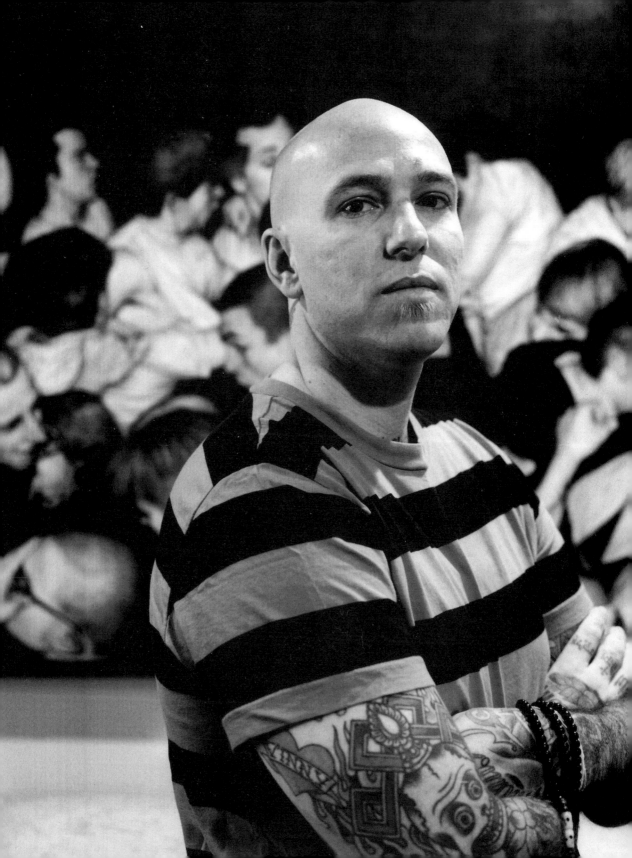

First published in Issue 21, Next Generation, Spring 2004

against the stream

punk, buddhism & the rebellion of waking up

[Noah Levine interviewed by John Malkin]

noah Levine has been going "against the stream" his whole life. Early on, punk rock mirrored his own desire to smash through personal and social patterns of ignorance and delusion. Later, Buddhism offered the internal tools to skillfully and gently engage in this upstream journey.

I invited Noah Levine to be a guest on the program I host on Free Radio Santa Cruz, a commercial-free, unlicensed radio station with roots in anarchist self-organization and nonviolent direct action. When I told Noah that I had interviewed a wide spectrum of people with views on social change and spiritual growth, from Vietnamese Buddhist monk Thich Nhat Hanh to Greg Graffin, lead singer of the punk rock band Bad Religion, Noah laughed and said, "Well, now you have both in one!" Mindfulness in the slam pit, anarchy laced with compassion. I was thrilled to find another person who loved punk rock and Buddhism, and to realize that there is a whole community of "dharma punx" out there just like me!

photo by David Black

Noah Levine is appealing to a new generation by blending the energy and action of punk with the wisdom and compassion of the Buddhist dharma. Punk rock and Buddhism share the fundamental philosophy that each of us creates our own reality. Real freedom is available as we learn to be aware in each moment, to take notice when we are caught in habitual streams of destructive thoughts or actions, and to experiment with consciously choosing to change those patterns.

In 500 BCE, the Buddha taught that any individual can wake up and be free from suffering; 2470 years later, the Sex Pistols proved that anyone could pick up a guitar and be in a band. The Buddha taught the importance of discovering the truth for one's self, through direct experience, not by simply taking someone else's word for it. The last teaching given by Buddha was, "Be a lamp unto yourself." A punk rock credo is "D.I.Y." – Do It Yourself.

In his recent book *Dharma Punx*, Noah Levine illustrates his own transformation from serving time in jail to serving others who are suffering in jails and prisons. He tells the stories of his life with an urgency that reveals his deep intention to be of service to those who are suffering, to bring Buddhist practices to young people who are struggling as he did.

Noah currently teaches meditation in juvenile halls and prisons around the San Francisco Bay Area and is director of the family program at Spirit Rock Meditation Center in California. The son of author and teacher Stephen Levine, Noah lives in San Francisco, where he is still deeply involved in the punk rock scene.

John Malkin   It is hard not to notice your arms and the artwork on your skin. You are covered in images of deities and spiritual teachers. Buddha, Krishna, Mary, Hanuman and Tara. Tell me about the tattoos on the tops of your hands that say "wisdom" and "compassion" with a lotus flower.

Noah Levine   A couple of years ago I was doing a long, silent meditation retreat at the Insight Meditation Society in Barre, Massachusetts. And during the retreat my mind was making its plans and fantasies and at one point during the retreat I had this vision of: "I want to get wisdom and compassion tattooed somewhere on my body." And since I already had sleeves and was pretty much covered in tattoos already, the tops of the hands were the optimal place, a very visual place to say, "This is what my intention for my life is and what my practice is. The cultivation of wisdom and compassion."

JM   You went through a lot to come to this place, where you are devoted to service and developing wisdom and compassion. How have Buddhism and punk rock come together in your life?

NL   The simplest way to explain it, for me, is that both are about the desire for happiness, the desire for freedom, and seeing the truth about life. As a kid I saw the truth about life. I was in a lot of pain and there was suffering everywhere. Inequality and oppression and war and racism. Capitalist-driven media crap. I just knew that happiness couldn't come from that.

My search for happiness, acceptance and freedom led me to punk rock. Punk had the energy, the information and the politics that I resonated with, but I took it to the nihilistic, self-destructive, drug-addicted, crime side of things. To that extreme. There definitely was an intense drive to escape from my own mind, from my emotions and my body. Drugs and alcohol offered that escape for a long time. To the point where I was so numb that I wasn't even aware of the crimes and the pain that I was causing myself and others. And on a whole other level I just didn't care, because I had really lost hope and wasn't able to take responsibility for my actions. There came a point where I was strung out and locked up and I had even lost my punk ethic in the pursuit of oblivion.

But that same energy of dissatisfaction and suffering eventually led me to start meditating while I was in prison. At the time, I thought that doing spiritual practice would be like completely fucking selling out. That was for hippies and that was for my parents and brain-dead religious followers. That was the masses to me. But I had lost all other hope. I felt like I had nowhere else to turn.

Meditation was a profound experience for me. I was able to just be present for that moment in my cell, rather than in the terror of prison and shame and regret for the crimes I had committed. I had been looking for that experience of freedom in punk and drugs and sex and crime, but I hadn't found it there, that real freedom.

JM   You wrote in Dharma Punx *that the spiritual path described by the Buddha is one of being against the stream, against selfish desires and ignorance and that "this fits in perfectly with the punk rock ethic."*

NL   Yeah. As I began to meditate and it really worked, I thought, "Actually, most people aren't doing this. This isn't mainstream! This isn't selling out. This is the punkest thing I've ever done." To learn to tell the truth after living a life of lies, to learn how to be kind to myself and to other people, that was the most rebellious and difficult action I have ever taken. This isn't buying in. This is waking up, waking up from this delusion that I have been in. And it is rebellious to do it.

I found a teaching where the Buddha said that practice is "against the stream," or an act of rebellion. Most people are suffering and don't even know it. They are so attached to pleasure and seeking pleasure all of the time that they will never wake up. So, I understood that teaching, because my whole life has been against the stream! There was a resonation, a deep knowing and reminder of something that I already knew. So I began integrating the punk ethic – that anti-establishment acknowledgement of suffering in the world – with the Buddhist philosophy that awakening, happiness and freedom are possible by acknowledging suffering and its causes, and cultivating awareness, morality and wisdom.

JM   Your father, Stephen Levine, is a prominent Buddhist teacher in America. Because he writes and teaches about healthy relationships, forgiveness, calmness and meditation, were there assumptions that he must have a happy family? Was this an extra burden you had to carry?

NL   Honestly, I didn't feel that pressure. On some level, I think it is the nature of children to rebel against their parents, so maybe there was some of that natural anti-parent rebellion going on. But I didn't really feel that. Really, I feel quite fortunate that I had this loving family. And on a whole other level, I may have had some karmic reincarnation. I might have come into this lifetime needing to exorcise these demons. I don't hold much blame. Actually, I am incredibly grateful that I had my father there when I was seventeen, to support and love and encourage me to quit fucking around and start practising.

JM   You were in jail and you got a phone call from your dad. He offered you meditation instructions over the phone and that was maybe the first time that you practised meditation, there in jail.

NL   Yeah. In a gentle and supportive way, he just said, "Look, what you're doing is just not working. Why don't you try something else?"

It was the first time that I ever meditated. I had been around it since I was a kid, but I'd never tried it. That was the turning point for me, of having the direct experience of it. I am a pessimist. I am skeptical about everything, so until I experience something for myself I think it's bullshit. And that was the first time I experienced it for myself. I was in enough pain that I was willing to even check out meditation. I thought, "Wow, this actually works to relax me a little bit. To calm me down a little bit." For a half a breath at a time. Not for hours. Not for days. But just for that moment of awareness. So I feel incredibly fortunate that I had my father on that level. There is a way in which it did save my life.

JM   You emphasize how important direct experience is for you. Tell me more about your experiences with meditation.

NL   My experience is that meditation develops slowly, over years. In no way is it a good time, all of the time. It is not like every time I meditate I feel great. What it is, is that every time I meditate I get in touch with the truth. And I am very interested in the truth. I get in touch with the truth of how distracted I am, of how crazy my mind is and how much pain my heart is in. I begin to take it all less personally. I understand how impermanent all phenomena are. And that I don't have to do anything, to push it away or hold onto it. And that when I do try to push it away or hold onto it, it creates this extra level of discomfort, of suffering, of dissatisfaction.

I certainly wasn't someone who came to meditation peaceful, looking for more peace. I came to it in tremendous suffering, looking for freedom. And I've found that. And it is not freedom from pain. It is freedom from identification. Freedom from the dissatisfaction that is inherent in trying to control the uncontrollable – the mind, the body, the world.

Meditation has, in my experience, led to an incredible sense that everything is unfolding in its own way. And I can have total intention without expectation on the outcome for my happiness. I can have full acceptance of what is happening in the present moment, with the intention to go somewhere else. Which I think is a huge, yet subtle distinction. People come to spiritual practice, and I have done this myself a lot, and say, "It's all about letting go, it's all about acceptance, so I just have to accept how fucked up everything is." But, it's more about how, "I don't accept how fucked up everything is and I want things to be better. I want to be happier, I want to be peaceful. I want to help other people."

JM   There is a lot of suffering in this world that needs to be addressed. There is sometimes the view that if you are "working on yourself" or developing spiritual practice, then you are not addressing the suffering of others.

NL   In my mind, they go hand in hand. I think that engaged action in the world is the total integral part of any spiritual practice. We have this vision of the Buddha as a renunciate. He was a renunciate, but he renounced greed, hatred and delusion. He renounced his possessions. But he stayed incredibly engaged in the societal issues of his times. He spoke out against racism and sexism, war, hatred and violence.

So, my practice arises simultaneously through the intention to purify my own mind and heart and to find freedom, along with the intention of discovering how I can use the freedom that I find to serve others. These two things have to be married, in my mind, in any kind of mature spiritual life.

The Buddha pointed out that there is suffering. This is the credo of punk rock. There is suffering and we don't like it: it sucks! The Buddha took it a step further and said, "Yes. And there is a cause of that suffering and there is a solution, an end to it, in the individual." Ultimately, I believe that there always has been and always will be corruption and suffering in the world. And I am not waiting for that corruption and suffering to end before I end my personal struggles. Punk made me aware of political injustice and Buddhism has taught me how to respond to it skillfully.

JM   Many people committed to spiritual practice struggle with the ideas of living as a monk versus staying in the world, or celibacy versus having a family. I wonder where you are at in that. And do you think that it is a struggle that can be resolved?

NL   At one point, I thought I would become a monk, but I just wasn't ready. Too much attachment, too much fear. Unresolved relationship issues in my life. So, I was in the monastery and it was just awful. It was painful to be there and not really be surrendered to being there. I may have been able to stick it out. I don't know. But I didn't.

I came home and felt very committed to being in the world and being of service. I started working in the jails and prisons, with my community and my generation. I thought, "This is it for me." But then a couple of years ago, when I was on a three-month retreat, about halfway through the retreat, I was really getting a deeper and deeper sense of my spiritual experience. My mind went totally toward monasticism. I felt, "This is so great. Why would I want to do anything else with the rest of my life? Why not just live in robes? How can I organize my life to live in robes and practise full-time?"

So, no, I don't think it is resolved within me. I will say that for the most part, I am leaning much more toward being a householder, living in the world, being in a relationship.

I would like to speak to this question on another level, too, though. On the level that we have in the West, this delusion of Buddhist practice, of spiritual practice, as needing to be one of pseudo-renunciation. We have this idea that if I am going to do spiritual practice, I need to live incredibly simply and I can't have money or nice things. I think that is really wrong. I have had that attitude a lot myself. One of my teachers told me recently that actually the Buddha said, "Renounce everything and become a monk or a nun, or if that is not your karma, if you're going to live in the world and be a householder, don't skimp to the point where you're struggling all of the time. Where you don't have anything extra to offer to anyone else."

I don't feel like I have all of the answers about this, but I feel pretty passionately that if you are not going to be a monastic and you're in the world, work! And do something that is of service to others. And use your life's energy to benefit other people. Use the money that you have in a skillful way. Don't think that you have to be broke. Love what you love. Have enough to share.

JM   I would like to hear briefly your story about meeting the Dalai Lama.

NL   He came to a meeting of all of the Buddhist teachers in the West in 2000 at Spirit Rock. I was there as Ram Dass's attendant, pushing him around in his wheelchair. You had to be teaching for ten years or something to be at the conference, so they kind of snuck me in as Dass's attendant.

One day, when the Dalai Lama was leaving the room after teaching, I was standing there and he was walking by blessing people that he came to and I was bowed, with my hands together in the prayer position. I was excited, knowing he was going to come and bow to me. And actually, when he approached me, he grabbed my hands in his and he saw the tattoo of Buddha and the tattoo of Krishna and Tara and some Tibetan images that I have and he looked right back into my eyes. My whole body was vibrating as he looked back at my arms and back up into my eyes and then he just says, "Very colourful!" And I just start cracking up. And everybody is cracking up and I am kind of, almost, leaving my body. It is just an overwhelming experience – the Dalai Lama is grabbing my arms and talking to me and making a joke about my tattoos. It was a powerful experience for me. Just a beautiful gift.

JM   Like you said, most people don't come to spiritual practice from a place of peace looking for more peace. Sometimes we have to face some very difficult things about ourselves. What would you say to young people who are starting to engage in some kind of practice?

NL   The Buddha said that this path is "against the stream." It is not natural. It's not easy. It takes tremendous effort and most people will never do it, because it is too subtle and difficult. But that is why we need to have the fellowship of the *sangha,* in the Buddhist term. Our generation has lived through the Cold War and Reaganomics and the birth, death and maybe rebirth of punk rock. To actually have a whole crew of punk rockers, or Generation Xers or Ys or whatever it is now…Wow!

There is something incredibly special about having a community of spiritual rebels. Spiritual revolutionaries. Being a punk rock Buddhist is really fucking lonely. I did it for ten years on my own. The only one, the only young person, the only tattooed person, the only punker at the meditation retreats. I wanted the teachings so bad that I didn't care. But I must admit that I do care! I love the fact that I have a community. That is why I wrote the book. To take the hippy, peace-loving stigma off of spiritual practice. To say that punks can do this. Punks maybe even have a head start because they understand suffering so well. Buddhist practice is simple, but it takes the courage of a warrior. ॐ

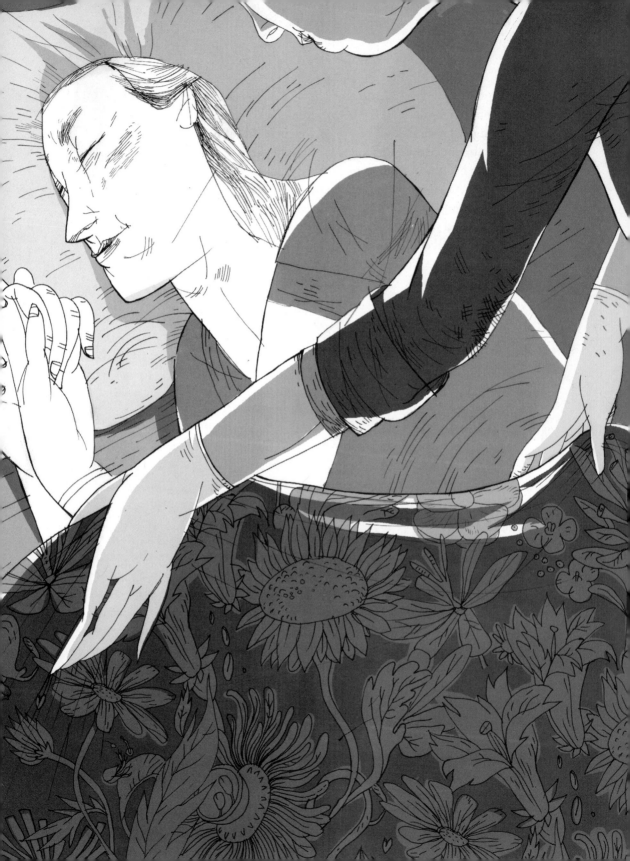

First published in Issue 23, Liberation, Fall 2004

feathers of regular moments
encountering daily saints

[by Gem Salsberg]

scalpel on peach flesh
the razor unzipping my belly
fingers reaching in to remove the poison pit
I was twenty-three years old. I had been volunteering, planting underwater eelgrass forests after a season of tree-planting. I've always been a woman of healthy appetite and vigorous constitution. It was strange when food began to repulse me. The light seemed different somehow, colder and more aquatic. The oddest pain began to flood me, a drowning spread of branching heat and black lattice-shaped shards. After many tests and the news that I had a tumour, I remember thinking, Is that how life works?

At first the words used to describe my flesh seemed cold and hard. *"The pancreas is a highly overengineered organ."* The tumour was possibly malignant and filled with carcinogenic fluids. If it leaked or ruptured, the poison would spread through my body. I lived with an unknown foreign bomb inside of me. I

illustration by Jillian Tamaki

began moving gently, cautious of the fragile egg perched on the cliff edge of my pancreas. My pancreas? A year before I would not have known what a pancreas does. Sometimes my body is unfamiliar, a separate creature with a city metropolis bustling and heaving inside a shell of skin.

let me tell you in simple talk

I had a tumour the size of a baseball on the end of my pancreas. My surgeon sliced me open, cut out the poison ball, stapled me up and plastic-wrapped me in morphine, codeine and blood thinners. I was in the hospital eleven days. The dietitian tried to feed me spaghetti and meatballs and chocolate ice cream. I wouldn't eat, only drank water. I wanted out of that raunchy illness-flushed death-smelling hospital with tortoise-armpit-green flasher gowns and pain like internal crucifixion (without any of the fiction).

Yet over and over grace arrived uninvited and unexpected, carried in the plain palms and feathers of regular moments.

A slender-necked pigeon flew to my window on the third-floor skyline. She was cramped on that windowsill. I had just opened my eyes for the first time and saw her. She looked in on me, turned her head, a side-crooked eye glance, then the other eye. I knew her. Messenger. I could close my eyes. And rest among the flaming horsetails and mad fiddlehead visions of stitch-ghosted hallways. The slanted crevice of Gravol and my electronic bed spun me beyond the edge of gravity.

awareness returning

My mother's voice was calling softly, "We're here. It's okay, Gemmy, we're here." Both eyes were swollen slits punching dim vision into a hard grey haze. Gauze wrapped my abdomen in a stiff muslin cocoon. My hand hovered below my heart, trying to speak. Nothing is real when pain is the singular encompassing experience. I heard voices, felt breath around me. This was real. This was comforting.

The first night, released of my humanness and magnified. Suffering so much that I could not speak past leaking, burnt coriander eyes silent. I lay curled and crying in a goose throat hollow pooled with salt.

janitor

She came from the shadow corridor. A woman in yellow gloves and rubber tongue squeaker shoes emerged through the eggplant crevice of middle night. A Filipina cleaning woman carrying holy water aqua green and spraying the acidic scent of false pine. She stopped, simply looked at me in the dark, a pause for pulse and breathing. After this subtle inhalation she pulled up a bucket and sat level to my damp sweating skull. She whispered,

"What you love?"

mountains birthed upwards around us
streams carved deep valleys and lakes gathered
the waters rose smooth and calm
a tinge of green edged the damp and gathered mineral to leaf
the slightest chance and trees carried the earth from darkness

All this revolved before I finally whispered a punctured word. "Garden."

She sat in the dark. Her head tilted, a soft lamplit child listening for the edge of clouds. Her canary rubber gloves began expressing the air in knuckle feathers, challenging my caves to become breathable. She told me of the fuchsia pallor of her petunias and the striated saffron sunburnt marigolds of her small backyard tendings. How mother deep her tangerine whispers of lush petunia growth, feather flashes of green arrows, crushed parsley stems and infant calendula cradles.

"Why the slugs eat all my nasturtiums?"

I understood then how simple life can be. It is real to care for someone who is in need, someone unknown, to risk the standard day for a life beyond basic survival.

She could have lost her job for stopping and being human. Bluebells and azaleas. Carrot weeds and roses. The green secrets of life bloomed in the air of my tunneled body cave and hushed out the flesh of her trowel-scented backyard.

a simple woman in such indigo shadow
i never saw her face

I was shocked. One morning I discovered that I had no care whether I lived or died. All the important heartbreaks and betrayals, the passions, hopes and motivated thrust of regular living evaporated. I discovered myself completely alone in a decreasing body. Breath became my companion.

Each night I lay awake and dreaming for the light to rise, for the mountains to swallow and digest me. I was flooded by an unfamiliar stillness. A single sunflower was left on my nightstand in a jar with sage and wild grass. I was okay, my mom was right. Okay even on this leaking raft of pain, on a heaving nauseation ocean. I was somehow more accepting and present than I had ever paused to actualize before.

Truth, a dawn of sunken marrow in my mind. The earth was being revealed again as precious. The kind of precious I had felt once when I lifted my tiny grandmother out of her wheelchair. Some determined god shouldered herself into my body and shouted at me, WAKE UP! But mostly she just whispered, *i love you, look how much i love you.*

a nurse
She tumbled the teal room alive under her chaos of gold-simmered hair, long labrador limbs and cheeks the shape of butter. She rag-dolled to my feet, paused and squinted some breathy curious smile. Then asked me a most unexpected question,

"Are you Dharma?"

I felt wrapped in burgundy. Saffron flooded my neck, ravens erupted from my knees and I thought, *how does she know, what i don't even know?*

She resembled the hue of pigeons and doves in her uniform under the diminishing dusk.

Many nurses and doctors came and went, checking and treating me. They each resonated a thriving core of care and intense devotion. One doctor was different. He was gruff and hard. I offered my hand, my name, hello. I was crying. I had just received the news that my first biopsy showed all the edge cells were healthy. I was crying for bright relief, crying for some strange mix of joy and sorrow, crying because I didn't even know what an edge cell was. I held up my palm on an unknown instinct. He wouldn't shake my hand or soften. He moved swiftly past to the chart of statistics at my feet and said, "Feeling a little emotional?" then left just as briskly.

erosion

He was so scared, so scared to love his patients. I wasn't insulted by him, I was revealed. My hand returned holding a space. I had known this space existed, but never had I fully embodied the bloom. Love. I simply felt such peace toward him. The ache I felt after he left the room was different from surgical pain. I felt sorrow for this man who was afraid to love. I felt how healing is an action of tenderness. The numbered patient is an echo waiting for response. My hand returned full, holding a teaching. All I need to do is place kindness out there, raise it up on the palm and offer this as a simple truth. Not everyone accepts the gift. I am alright with this. Sometimes the real healing is deeper than the body, than all its limbed and porous crevices. Healing smooths out the fissures of the damaged sandstone soul.

Liberation is not a holy blessed brilliant lightning bolt explosive divine angel choir glowing virginal palms pierced levitating suffering illusionary perfect pristine glorious bright pearly toothed god-human. LIBERATION is the janitor. Yes, that Filipina woman in stretched-too-tight gloves with a bottle of cleaning chemicals and a cart of plastic hygiene. The woman who stopped in a room at 3 a.m. where this woman called "me" was leaking silent tears and fluids.

see how precious this brief life is, every single breath is precious

I saw how I bring nothing tangible into this world. Nothing that flesh will retain, nor wood nor pebble, green creature or lidded. Paint crumbles away over aged paper deserts and slowly my body becomes driftwood, leaning in on silver skin.

Surgery carved out a tumour but something else was left inside. Fresh space, potential space. Space for rent. Somehow all life became so ordinary. The kind of ordinary that is parsnip beautiful, the kind of ordinary that wrenches all wants and grudges and castanet dreams and flips them inside out like grandmother's pink-petaled pillowcases. Surgery sliced the extraneous searching and cut me to the essential question. Why am I here? What is the purpose I was born for?

Here I am, under my skin. It has been over a year and a half. There's a very large and beautiful pink-ridged scar on my belly in the shape of an L.

listen, listen here

I hear an undercurrent, a hum. I have heard the healing mantra in bus wheels and diesel fumes, in rose hedges and door hinges, in the voice of a woman outside the grocery store asking for spare change. Lost in the common sacred day the moons rise on each of my toes. I am a planet in this quick galaxy. I am so vast. I am so small. This is revealed to me by daily saints and common people living basic real lives. Practising compassion in their unassuming way and showing how essential it is to breathe and be grateful, love and be grateful, try and be grateful. The teachings of each day are modest and mostly silent.

There are rust-orange butterflies above me when gazing gently. Every person and each cold-brimmed house becomes a home, a neighbour, a possibility for me to learn to love. To love as a moth seeking light in every acrid flickering body. Love as a brilliant instinct, an insect surging toward the need, the porch-light beacon. Love as the ability to not take personally injured action as an affront but to see with seven thousand fractalled eyes, each harmed action as a cry out, a vivid yearning for a mother's patience.

messenger

I taught my first Hatha Yoga class this morning, was nervous and wondering, What do I have to offer? Heard a tap tap tapping at the window. Everyone paused their poses. I turned and saw her looking through the glass. A little acorn-shaped bird. Charcoal storm cotton, she was a puff of smoke feathers. Checking in on me, through one eye and then the other.

Cupped hand, offering.

i love you, look how much i love you. ॐ

All healing is the work of love, because all healing takes place in a context where we wish to promote growth ... Any time people are genuinely engaged in a practice of healing, it brings them into greater community with others.

First published in Issue 24, Health & Healing, Winter 2004

the ingredients of love

love & healing as political resistance

[bell hooks interviewed by Juniper Glass]

b ell hooks is fascinated by love. For years, she has looked at love from all directions, and in the course of all this seeking discovered a contradiction in our understanding of love.

"Everywhere we learn that love is important, and yet we are bombarded by its failure," she writes in *All About Love: New Visions*. "Awesomely, our culture is driven by the quest to love even as it offers so little opportunity for us to understand love's meaning or to know how to realize love in word and deed…. We see little indication that love informs decisions, strengthens our understanding of community, or keeps us together."

A writer, teacher and cultural critic, bell hooks is best known for her work examining systems of domination, especially racism and patriarchy, and how they may be overcome. She has published more than twenty books, including *Talking Back: Thinking Feminist, Thinking Black; Killing Rage: Ending Racism;* and *Where We Stand: Class Matters*. hooks says that uncovering and naming the forms of oppression in our society is an extension of her lifelong curiosity about love and her desire to see love manifested.

"Perhaps the most common false assumption about love is that it means we will not be challenged or changed," she once wrote in the Buddhist magazine *Shambhala Sun*. "When I write provocative social and cultural criticism that causes readers to stretch their minds, to think beyond set paradigms, I think of that work as love in action. While it may challenge, disturb and at times even frighten or enrage readers, love is always the place where I begin and end."

Like Martin Luther King, one of her key sources of inspiration, hooks believes that love is a path that can end violence and injustice and heal the wounds of oppression. But walking this path requires much more than the wish, "Can't we all love one another?" Love isn't a feeling that just happens, hooks says, it is a choice and an action that must be practised in our everyday lives, as "the will to nurture another's spiritual growth or one's own."

I spoke with hooks by telephone while she was in Toronto on a lecture tour. She was delighted to focus the conversation on healing and brought her characteristic straight-talking, deep-thinking approach to the subject. She calls attention to the misconceptions about the healing process; it doesn't mean perfection or freedom from pain, but rather growing up, overcoming self-centredness and entering into greater community with others.

Born Gloria Watkins in small-town Kentucky, she chose the pen name bell hooks in honour of a female ancestor with a reputation for speaking her mind. I expected hooks, a former professor at Yale and one of America's leading public intellectuals according to the *Atlantic Monthly*, to speak with the fierceness I have sometimes read in her books. Her voice, however, was profoundly sweet and warm. Her statements often ended with an open lilt, not the kind that sounds like a question mark, expressing uncertainty, but instead full of curiosity, inviting me to wonder and explore along with her.

Juniper Glass How would you define love?

bell hooks Love is a combination of six ingredients: care, commitment, knowledge, responsibility, respect and trust. I found that a lot of people just felt really confused about what love is, so I said, here, take these six ingredients and as you go about your life, you can ask: the action I'm taking, does it have these six ingredients?

One point that I would emphasize to people is that it's the combination of the six ingredients that make love, because so many of us have one of the ingredients in our life – like we may be deeply cared for, but we may not be in a situation of trust. To me what's great about these definitions is that they're just very helpful for people in daily life trying to engage in a practice of love.

JG   What is the link between healing and loving?

bh   Well, it seems to me that all healing is the work of love, because all healing takes place in a context where we wish to promote growth. We wish to engage the organism in ways that people grow stronger. I find myself telling people that my wish for the rest of my life is that all the work I do would be about healing. I want people to heal. My concern is always to link those practices of healing with practices of political resistance.

JG   What needs to be healed? Is it the heart, the mind, the spirit?

bh   For many of us, whether it's turning toward Buddhism, or like many African American people who have turned toward Yoruba, the healing is a healing into wholeness, moving away from the sense of the self as splintered and fractured and broken. But it's not a healing into perfection. It's not a vision of wholeness that says everything will become right with me. It's an acceptance that says we are, at our core, essentially whole even in the midst of our flaws and our woundedness. And it's an acceptance that includes those flaws and wounds and that includes the embrace of pain.

I think particularly in the Western world, and in the United States especially, people have a vision of healing that is about feeling that you must be free from pain. Other than a vision of healing that says we can restore a sense of balance to our being that may allow us to cope with pain in ways that are restorative. So pain isn't perceived as the enemy but as the point of possibility and transformation.

I think that vision is really hard to keep alive in a culture that's always offering people some kind of drug that promises to take the pain away. So many people I talk to, young people who are lusting for wealth, imagine that there's some wealth they will achieve that will take pain away in their lives. No matter how much we hear from people who have great wealth about the pain in their lives, people continue to maintain this fiction.

JG   Do you think that everyone has something that needs to be healed?

bh   No. I think that almost every person will encounter some physical ailments in their lifetime (but we also know that the body is capable of such enormous and profound spontaneous healing). Some people like to say to me, "Oh, doesn't everybody come from a dysfunctional family?" And they get really annoyed when I say, "Well, no, I don't think so." I think there are very, very lucky individuals who've come from functional families. But I think that because those of us from dysfunctional families are more the norm in a sense, more common, it's easy to overlook the powers of people coming from caring, loving, functional families.

JG   Healing implies that something is broken. How can we keep from seeing ourselves too much as victims during the healing process?

bh   I think that in a culture like the West that values youth and power so much, the whole idea of being flawed in any way often leads people to embrace victimhood, whether people think they're flawed in the space of race or flawed in the space of gender. And I think the difference between a healing approach that leads to greater empowerment of self and one that leads to greater diminishment of self is that it's all about accountability. There isn't any need to posit blame. I think at the core of any embrace of victimhood is the will to blame and to feel as though something outside of ourselves that we can't control is acting upon us in some way that renders us powerless.

JG   One of the ideas I like in your writing is that healing is essentially a growing-up process. It involves taking full responsibility for our lives.

bh   Exactly. And I think that has to be viewed, in the context of the West, as a project of political resistance because there's so much in the daily-ness of our lives that militates against a vision of growing up. I think that we live in the ultimate Me culture, where everything is always brought back to that sense that the ego or the self is at the centre and what matters most. Sometimes as a teacher I laugh and tell my students, "You know everything is not about you!" And there are days in my life when I have to remind myself that everything is not about me!

JG   You say that "serving others is as fruitful a path to the heart as any other therapeutic practice."

bh   Like Thich Nhat Hanh says you can heal anything with the breath, I think that service to others is a kind of symbolic breath you take. It takes you away from the very I-centredness we're talking about. Service is that wonderful spiritual practice we can do daily.

JG   And also, when we take action it increases our sense of empowerment. When we make a small act, it isn't a revolutionary change, but then the feeling of empowerment grows.

bh   Yes. I remember saying that statement in church all the time, "I cannot do everything but I can do something. God help me, I will do." A lot of the work that I'm doing, I'm trying to address the trauma felt by many people who have experienced race or gender forms of oppression. But I'm also trying to not just fixate on the experience of trauma but to embrace the agency of healing. When we become so fixated on what we feel someone has done to us, whether it's group oppression or individual oppression, we can get stuck in the naming of that pain. It's a certain kind of soaking in that pain that becomes an identity rather than moving through into greater awareness.

Many people of colour ask me: Well, aren't you concerned that people will focus on individual healing and won't be concerned with projects of collective resistance? And my response is, and I make this comment a great deal, I feel that healing never takes place in the context of aloneness. Any time people are genuinely engaged in a practice of healing, it brings them into greater community with others.

JG How did you encounter a spiritual path?

bh   I started out as very much in the fundamentalist Baptist church of the south. When I went away to college I was very interested in the Beat poets and that led me to Buddhism, particularly fellowshipping with Gary Snyder when I was seventeen and eighteen years old. My own love of poetry has been the vehicle that has awakened me to greater awarenesses of different faiths. Poetry has been the path that has led me to Islamic mysticism, to Kabir and Rumi back in the days when they weren't commonplace names.

Every day I have a meditation and just this morning I was meditating on poetry by the Sufi mystic Ibn Arabi. He says, "I profess the religion of love wherever its caravan turns. Along the way that is the belief, the faith I keep." And that's often how I see myself. I sometimes joke that I'm the high priestess of love! I see myself as this person on a journey of love whose task it is to create a body of work that leads people into greater love, which means for me into greater care, commitment, knowledge, respect, with themselves and others. I think that that is the healing of self and communities. ॐ

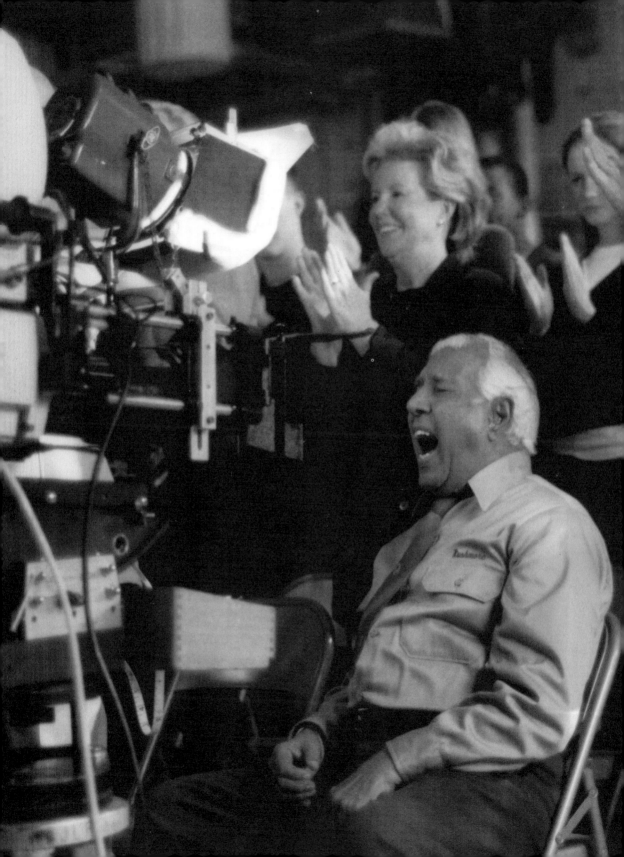

First published in Issue 23, Liberation, Fall 2004

kumar

the secret teachings of kumar pallana

[by Jeffry Farrell]

(1)

Kumar, this is J.

Hello, man. How're you?

I'm in Paris.

Oh, man, what are you doing in Paris?

Well, I've been making theatre and studying and teaching …

Are you divorced yet?

Yeah. Yes. Legally.

How's the kid?

She's alright … She's with …

You must come live with me, man.

What? What are you talking about? Kumar. I can't *live* with you.

Oh no, you don't know what you are saying. You must come live with me, man.

photo courtesy of Jeffry Farrell

Stay with me. We'll work out, eat, practise yoga. You'll see. Where else is your plan, man?

I don't think Dallas is the best place for me to …

Not Dallas, man. Come stay with me.

Where?

In Dallas, man. With me. When you come, you will see, you will see it is your best choice. Loves you, goodbye.

Click.

(2)

Months later, exhausted and sweating, I drive up to Kumar's garage apartment behind his café, the Cosmic Cup. I park and go up the garage apartment's steps. Across the gravel a speaker sounds a raga from under the Cup's eaves. I want nothing, maybe relief.

Kumar is not due back from India for a couple of days. I enter the apartment – a refuge of cardamom air and solitude. The window unit blows cool. I stand there, my face in the A/C. I turn to the open room: two windows shaded with blinds reveal a floor of worn, rose-colored carpet, a single bed in the far corner, a green leather chair, a TV, bookcases laden with books and Hindu icons, a crack in the cinder block wall clear through to the outside. On the wall hangs a bas relief golden Ganesh (plastic), images of a blue Krishna in a forest, of Jesus in the garden, of Vivekenanda standing, arms crossed. There's a poster of yoga poses and photos of Kumar performing in Las Vegas, Los Angeles, New York, Paris.

Twinkle lights blink outside the window blinds. The raga never ends. I fall asleep on the carpet.

In daylight I wash piled, crusty dishes and dry them. I rub out the sink, stove and floor. In the fridge I find eggs dated from two months ago, hard bread, green sour cream, a partial gallon of congealed milk and yogurt tubs of repellent odour. I take out the garbage. I wipe the bathroom's shower, toilet, mirror and basin. I wash my clothes and the bedclothes in the Cosmic Cup's washer upstairs. I buy milk and bread, eggs and rice to replace what I'd thrown away.

(3)

Kumar arrives late in the evening. The twinkle lights blink. The raga sounds. Kumar comes in coughing. He drops his bag. Is he choking? He waves a feeble hello and gives me a hug. He lifts birdseed from a bookcase shelf, pours the seed on an aluminum plate and places the plate outside the door. He comes in and lies down on his bed. He looks really old, lying on his side, looking at me. He coughs and says.

I have the coughing.

What from?

It's the dust. India.

Do you need medicine?

Just rest it. We'll talk tomorrow. Can you bring me a glass of water?

Twinkle lights blink and the raga continues. Kumar coughs all night. I have a sleeping mat and blanket on the rose-coloured carpet. Possibilities pass through my mind. It starts to rain. Kumar's coughing abates. I fall asleep.

(4)

Kumar shows me how to make his chai. He boils the tea until it spills over onto the stovetop. He curses and we laugh.

We sit at his deuce-top table in metal diner chairs. We catch up with stories and chai.

We move onto the open floor. We warm up. He leads me through a series of *asanas,* and finally directs my right hand to cup the carpet, my left hand to take my left ankle and lift high behind me. My eyes fix on a woven carpet loop. I balance on my right foot. Kumar says, "Hold it. Don't let go. Hold it. Put your soul into it …"

When I let go, I fall from a cliff. I collapse to the ground.

"Other side. Go! Hold it. Breathe! Go man! Put your soul into it!"

I hold it. I fall from a second cliff.

Thomas Merton has written that "in silence we face and admit that gap between the depths of our being, which we consistently ignore, and the surface which is so often untrue to our own reality." My depth and my surface merge.

I lie in silence on the rose-coloured carpet. I cannot move. Nothing to say; I have no thoughts. Kumar says, "Enough."

(5)

From the attic of the Cup, I retrieve juggling rings, bags of performance plates and the plate-spinning tables – all handmade and handpainted. These remain intact from Kumar's performing days. Kumar and I settle into an improvised routine of Hatha practice, *pranayam, kriya* and meditation, cooking, resting, balancing, juggling and rope tricks. When not with Kumar, I teach part-time.

On Saturday nights we watch Wrestlemania and the Big Shot westerns. To prepare, I clean and cut spinach, potatoes, tomato, onion, cilantro, ginger. Kumar cooks. He makes kitcheree, parotas and pakora, and we eat. We drink Crown Royal and Coke or Meyers dark rum and Coke, over ice. Kumar sits in his green chair munching Lays potato chips. He rubs his finger between dentures and gum to retrieve loose chip fragments. I balance red and white hoops on my forehead during commercials. The movie comes back on.

That's going to be you and me, man. Everyone will watch us on Saturday night. You wait, I means it, you'll see.

Kumar, what kind of yoga are you teaching me?

Don't you know by now it's all yoga? Clint Eastwood, man, he's great. *Sierra Madre* is next.

Oh man, Bogart. He's the great, too.

(6)

Upside-down in a handstand, my wrists trouble me.

Kumar says, Don't force it, man.

What?

Look at your hands, man. No, no, turn them out more. There. Wide fingers. Wide. Put your soul into it. That's it! Feel the difference? This protects your wrists.

I come down to rest on my knees: Kumar! I've been practising with you for how long? And now you tell me my wrists have been wrong! I could have avoided the injury in my wrists, which has been the trouble with my handstands all this time!

Look, man. If I tell you everythings, what good is that? You never really learn. It comes and it goes. Really learn. Look at nature. That's the teacher. Practise. That's the teacher. Learn. Look at the birds. Do they say, I will do this ten times or twenty? Do they try? No. Look how they come. They have their order. They have their way. No one teaches them. Be practicals. I am not teaching you the common way, not from any books. I am teaching you the step way. This is not about ego. This is about getting the grip. Yoga is the creation, not just this routine or that ones, not the *asanas*. You see with the grip, then more and more. No shortcuts, man.

(7)

We live in a universe complementary to the city of Dallas. We live with one foot in the mundane and the other foot in a landscape of continuous creation. While everyone hustles and bustles, Kumar and I live behind the Cosmic Cup. My speech with him begins to reflect Kumar's accent although we don't need many words between us. I see my daughter, who tells me my body smells of curry. Kumar tells me that he wants to teach me everything he knows before he dies ...

What?

Just listen.

What?

Listen. You ask me what kind of yoga. It's all yoga – the Hatha, the Karma, the *kriya*, the *bhakti*, the *raj*, everything – the cooking, the breathing, the story. Yoga is the creative expression. This is my style. It's the union. Look around you, everything once was first the thought: this table, this room, this building, the street, the cars, everything, even the trees and the birds. Someone had to think it.

My point is – the thought is powerful, the most powerful thing. Observe the thought forms. Don't waste it with worry. This is number one. Second, money. It comes and it goes. What you need it for? You have survived all this time without any more, and your daughter, too. Her mother has the good job. Be practicals. You don't really need. You will survive. She will survive. So many people around the world, they don't have. They survives. But so, even you don't have it, that's good, too, man. That means it's coming. You'll see. And third, so you get the money. Where is the end? How much is enough? Be happy with what you have no matter what you have. Be simple. Like me. Look at the very rich man. He is more worried than you. Someone is going to takes it, he is going to lose it, all these things. Be the same however you are, rich or poor. Remember this, what I'm saying. Write it down.

(8)

I drive Kumar to his doctor's appointments. I drive him to the social security offices, to the Dallas county tax office, to daily appointments, to the AAA road club office. Kumar introduces me as his son. Students come and go. Kumar has me demonstrate. We begin to travel.

I'm driving on the interstate somewhere east of New Orleans. Kumar lifts his face.

You know, I meditate so that I can die. Every time is a practice.

(9)

Kumar's feet are ugly. They itch and trouble him. His toenails are crusty with fungus. I buy a gallon of bleach, a box of foot-soaking powder and some herbs. I fill a tub with warm water and add bleach. I place a white towel on the floor under Kumar's green chair. As we watch Hulk Hogan and company, Kumar soaks his feet. I balance two rings on my forehead. At a commercial, I remove the tub, take clippers and begin to trim every encrusted, octogenarian toenail. It is less work to trim a hedge of briar. I return his feet to soak in a tub of herbs. I clean up. We drink rum and Coke.

You have to teach, man.

I teach, Kumar – high school, college.

You have the full-time? The benefits?

No.

You have to teach the yoga.

Mmm …

You have to, man. Why not? You know more than these peoples who go to California and get the paper and boom they are yoga teachers.

What do I know about yoga? I teach theatre, mime, acting. I'm not a yoga teacher.

Have the confidence, man. Every dog has his bite. Teach my students. Talk to them. Let them come.

Yeah. Okay, if you say so.

Yes, I say so. The fact is there.

(10)

Years pass. In my kitchen, I wash dishes after midnight. The phone rings and I catch it before it wakes the children. Kumar's nocturnal voice is a shout of birds in the rain.

Kumar!

How're you, man?

I go out to the garage and get inside my Jeep. Except for the phone receiver's light, it is completely dark.

Kumar. Fill me in. Are you in Paris?

I'm still in India. They loves me, man. I could stay here as long as I want, but I am making the TV pilot in Los Angeles in two weeks. We have the good actors and writers. And it is paying me good money by the week. But you know if nothing happens I am happy. I have my share. God is good to me. And I have to ask – what good is any of this to me now? I am old, man. If this happened thirty years ago, then that would be something, then you'd really see something. I really, really means it. What good is any of this? I came nude and I goes out nude. The fact is there. Maybe I'll go out in the jungle. Nobody knows. How're you, man?

I'm alright. Working too much, but you know I have the children. I have some worries.

You have to stop that, man. You should know by now, stop the worry. You're a teacher. Every kid has his own destiny, his own luck. And somebody has to bring them into this world. That's your luck! You have to start laughing, just laugh. You know, nobody knows, but the *mala* is helping me, man. I am practising the breath and the rhythm. The rhythm is everything. This is helping me more than anything. Not ten times, not hundred times, but hundreds and hundreds. That's the secret. Practice.

When you practise you find the honesty in the thought form. Honest have to be perfect honest, not a little greedy. It's a surrender. That's how the peace comes. Any thought form you have, any clear desire you create must be pure. Must be a surrender. You have a nice milk and you see what comes when you put one drop lemon. See what comes.

Kumar laughs. ॐ

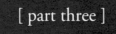[part three]

reflection / encounters with self

Self-study, inner work and reflection are at the heart of yoga. With the deepest respect, *ascent* allows its writers to open their lives to the page, to all of us. The intimate is revealed, the doubt and pain, the strength and bliss. In spiritual life, we meet ourselves. This is never an easy encounter, but it can be poetic, funny, beautiful, sad and always worthwhile. *ascent's* dedication to inquiry and self-discovery is practised in its pages. The authors pursue the meaning of yoga. Perhaps there are not solid answers, but sometimes it is the sincerity of questioning that is important.

In her essay "17 Hours in China" Sarah E. Truman concludes: "I'm alone, listening to the wind in the bamboo behind the empty Guan Yin temple. I know what it means. I don't know what it means…"

This is how *ascent* shines. These are inspired lives.

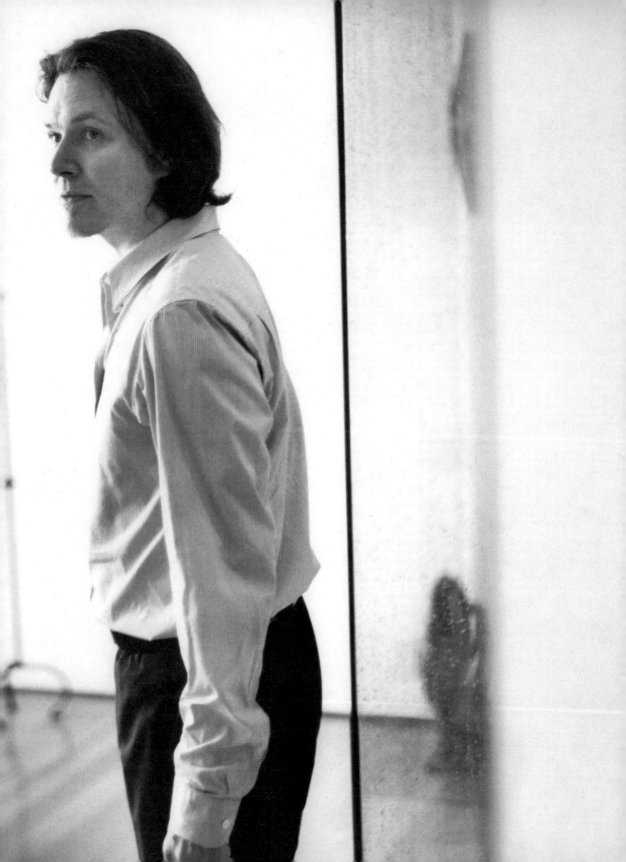

First published in Issue 23, Liberation, Fall 2004

blemish

embracing the complexities of *sadhana*

[David Sylvian interviewed by Marcus Boon]

my favourite David Sylvian song is called "Fire in the Forest." Recorded in 2003 for his recent CD, *Blemish,* the song, just a voice singing over a humming guitar drone, has a gentle intensity that pulled me through a winter spent riding around on public transportation in the suburbs of Toronto. Phrases such as "there is always sunshine/ behind the grey skies/ I will try to find it/ yes I will try" heard on headphones again and again in snowy darkness somehow showed a fragile determination to transcend the ego's limits. The track itself is all the more moving for its place at the end of a record full of dark songs about spiritual struggle.

Blemish is not a word normally associated with spiritual practice, yet the record reflects Sylvian's growing and deepening experience of *sadhana,* first with Mother Mira, then Shree Ma, with whom Sylvian and his family lived in California in the mid-1990s, and in recent years with Mata Amritanandamayi or Ammachi, as she's affectionately known.

photo by Darren Keith

Sylvian grew up in a non-religious family in South London, England and formed the group Japan in 1974. The group went on to considerable success as glam/new romantic rockers, but broke up after releasing the marvelous *Tin Drum* (1981). Sylvian has pursued a solo career since, with early highlights including *Brilliant Trees* (1983) and *Secrets of the Beehive* (1987). A master of material describing an existential spiritual struggle – such as *Tin Drum*'s "Ghosts" with its chorus, "Just when I think I'm winning/ when I've broken every door/ the ghosts of my life/ blow wilder than before" – Sylvian's songs have taken on an increasingly explicit spiritual form, reflecting his studies with various teachers after his move to America in the 1990s, where he still lives with his wife, singer Ingrid Chavez, and children.

After the devotional lushness of 1999's *Dead Bees on a Cake*, the austere, intense *Blemish*, with its stunning minimalist guitar work courtesy of Christian Fennesz and Derek Bailey, comes as a surprise. The surprise for me, however, is one of recognition, of having feelings, confusions and internal struggles that I could not find a way of articulating suddenly manifested, in gentle yet rigorous form.

One of Sylvian's most remarkable songs, *Secrets of the Beehive*'s "Orpheus," sings of the Greek legend, whose singing could charm animals, humans and gods alike. We think of music today as something disposable, as "pop," as background music. Without hiding behind the rhetoric of "high art" or of any particular religious practice, Sylvian's music points to that Orphic power of music, to reveal to ourselves what it means to be alive.

I met Sylvian in downtown Manhattan with his ten-year-old daughter, Amira. The singer still has the beauty of legend, but little of the ethereal quality that is habitually attributed to him. He speaks quietly, thoughtfully, precisely, while his daughter speaks on a cellphone to her mother, or lounges, reading, generously tolerating us.

David Sylvian   I often feel that there's a greater union between myself and my teacher when I'm not physically in their presence. There's a whole other level of experience when I'm in their presence, but that sense of non-physical merging, of intimacy, is profound.

Marcus Boon It's surprising that you can visit someone who's been dead for 600 years and burst into tears in their presence. That's how I felt at Hazrat Allaudin Sabri's shrine in India. They say that he was so fierce in his lifetime that the only person who could come physically close to him was a musician, who would sit fifty feet away and play for him. And you can still feel that fierceness today!

DS That's another element, isn't it? The element of ferocity in the proximity of the guru. People talk about the experience of bliss, but the level of ferocity, the fire that one has to walk through, live through – that is also very intense. The degree of suffering increases as the experience of *sadhana* deepens, for me, because at first there's less attachment to who one believes one is and it's easier to let go of all the things that need to be let go of. As you move through different stages, the degree of fear increases because ultimately you're getting to the root foundations of the ego, which are unshakeable. And there is real fear because you see the death of the ego approaching, and if you let go of that, what is there?

As you have to face your fears in the presence of your guru, you witness other people going through their experiences. There's often this perception, "Why do I have to live through this fear? I'll take on anybody else's obstacles, but not this one!" [laughs]. It's so pinpoint-perfect, it's precision-made, this laser-like intensity focusing on just what needs to be focused on. Once you move beyond a given level of fear, apprehension, there's an enormous release and a whole new world of possibility seems to open up. You live and breathe that for a while until you come up against that next obstacle.

MB A lot of people like to think that a spiritual narrative consists in going from darkness and suffering to peace and equanimity, but I think of your music, and in particular of Blemish, *which is so much darker than the records that came before. It's still a record about* sadhana …

DS It's darker than ever! But going through that experience of darkness at this point in my life was very different to before. First of all, there was a certain amount of objectivity, of being able to step back and say, all of this is just par for the course, it's just part of the learning process, whatever comes out of this is just to strengthen me and help me to burn off whatever needs to be cleared away so that I can see things clearly.

And a lot of things that I couldn't face in my life I could face in the studio environment. I would close that door and start working and open myself to whatever came through. And often it was very negative emotions. And I thought, well, I'll just look straight at them, and more than that, I'll take them even further than I feel them in my daily life, because I wanted to go as far with them as I possibly could. I felt very safe doing that. I felt that there was a strength inside of me that would allow me to pull back at the end of the day and be able to do away with those emotions. So I was pushing myself deeper and deeper into the negativity of the experience, wanting to know what that felt like, how does that surface and how do you give that a voice? It was a way of experiencing those experiences and giving them a new vocabulary that was pertinent for now.

MB   Now, as in our time?

DS   Yes. I was also feeling that all the familiar forms of popular song were no longer doing it for me. Even those evergreen artists that you go back to time and time again weren't moving me anymore. The form had lost its potency; it had been exhausted. I was beginning to feel: What next? What do you do? And I felt that I personally had to find a new form for what I was experiencing. I feel it's true of other arts, too: now is an important time to find vocabularies that are pertinent to our time.

Everything becomes a commodity. We're told that if we understand someone's taste in how they decorate their home, then we can probably guess what kind of music will go with that environment. Everything gets tied together in packages so we can all have what's known as "good taste." We can dress well, we have good taste in our cultural environment, we can participate in it but without any commitment, no going out on a limb, always tapping into something that's termed "classic," whether it's a couch or a Marvin Gaye record.

But when we find something that challenges all of that in the culture, that's when we discover who we are, and our response isn't preconditioned. We don't have the benefit of reading a review of this experience prior to having it. We have to comprehend it on our own terms, ask: "Why did I feel so irritated when I was provoked in that way?" I want to have that kind of experience. The one that isn't scripted. The one that will throw you into the deep end of an experience and you just have to work it out for yourself. There is no right or wrong response, only your true response. And that's what I try to find in my work, that true response. It doesn't necessarily make it that comfortable an experience to listen to, but that's not the issue here. It's just trying to find a means to grapple with what it means to be alive in the here and now, trying to find a vocabulary for it, trying to press the right buttons in me, and hopefully that will communicate to others.

MB   When you think of musicians who've become involved in sadhana, *they often take on the costumery that comes with* sadhana, *but you seem to have made a conscious decision against doing that …*

DS   It's just not an outfit that feels comfortable to wear. You try everything at some point or another. When I was with Shree Ma we went through that, as a family, supporting and performing with her, but it didn't feel right.

MB   Have you done bhajans?

DS   I haven't recorded them, but we've sung them, obviously. I'm very familiar with the form. But there's a certain resistance to that as a musician, an artist. I feel that I'm a very fallible person, I have powerfully conflicting emotions, and I don't want to give the false impression that all is right in my world.

On one level, the world has a beautiful simplicity and clarity to it; on another level it's only got far more complicated, with an increased degree of suffering. Sometimes I may only want to focus on the blissful elements of Divine awareness, maybe within an entire project or just within one piece of music. Or maybe it lies behind everything I do already. It's hard to say. I don't analyze what I do to that degree. But I can't do away with all the questions I have about what it means to be alive in the here and now, all the troubles and emotional conflicts, the love and hate that live side by side.

I don't believe I ever feel only love except possibly in the lap of Amma. Outside of that beautiful place, love is accompanied by a whole complexity of emotions, including its mirror opposite. I want my work to have that complexity, because the best work is the kind of material that, no matter what frame of mind you come to it with, you can still see yourself mirrored in it.

The great failure of so-called "spiritual music" that we're surrounded by in this culture is that it's a music that tries to placate, it tries to insist that you be peaceful and filled with love. Well, nothing could irritate me more than being surrounded by a work of art at any level that insists I feel something. I would rather my work embody all the possibilities and let people find themselves within it, and find a release. That's the best that I can do. I wouldn't want to give the impression of an ivory tower existence where nothing seems to touch you anymore, that somehow you can ride over all these obstacles because you've found a greater inner peace.

MB That's the problem of New Age music, and why so many people are so resistant to the idea of spiritual practice, or music that addresses spiritual issues.

DS Yes, but it's funny... We spoke earlier about spiritual music, and the first name that came up was John Coltrane. And that's the antithesis of everything we think of culturally as spiritual music. But it's right there, the fire of purification, of suffering, of bliss. It's all there, embodied, and you can tap into that work on any of those fundamental levels and experience it in a beautiful and profound way. That's the beauty and strength of a work that reflects all that we are and potentially can be. Maybe it's too much to strive for and maybe you're guaranteed to fail 99.9 percent of the time. But it's definitely a goal worth aspiring to.

MB Your own sadhana *is involved in very complex spiritual traditions, but the terms in which you describe spiritual struggle in your music, aside from a song like "Krishna Blue" on* Dead Bees on a Cake, *avoid direct reference to these traditions and practices. Why do you think that is?*

DS I don't want to fall into a stereotypical response to my relationship to the

Divine. I don't want it to feel too comfortable in my own work, as a writer. Writing a piece like "Krishna Blue" – that was during a period of the enormous romance of the relationship with the guru, which is lovely, and it's still present in my life. But now I want to deal with the complexity.

In a sense, the guru romances you to begin, you kind of get an easy ride so that you can just experience all the profound love that is there, without the discoloration of your own ego. And once you have been led in so far, you begin to have experiences that are more profound but far more difficult to undergo. I don't want to fall back on the romance of the journey. What is more intriguing is the reality of the journey because the reality is so much more amazing than simply the romance. The reality of the journey encompasses so much, and there's no separation from it in any aspect of life. Not one aspect, no matter what one is doing. That's an incredible thought.

I compartmentalized my life at some point, saying, there's this and there's that and then there's spiritual life. To me, now, it's all become spiritual life. Compartmentalizing seems to be borne out of what one perceives to be the good and bad in one's self, the different faces we show to ourselves, and ultimately the need to tell a story about who we are that excludes activities that don't quite fit in with the story, which we may enact occasionally and then bury when they're no longer necessary. There's no part I'll allow myself to push to one side and say, well, that's my dirty little secret and I keep that over there. No, it's all a part of my spiritual life. That's a tremendous recognition. Years and years of analysis couldn't have brought me to this point in time, to bring all of these separate elements together and embrace them as one.

MB It's so hard to know what to do with the outbursts, the things that one would like to be exceptions to the nice pure spiritual system. I love that title, Blemish, *for that reason. It's the hardest thing to face up to.*

DS It really is. To me the notion of telling a story about who one is, while it facilitates a sense of mental well-being and coherence to one's life journey, is basically a lie. It's so well edited that it can't possibly embrace who we really are, and of course who we really are is beyond all of that. So I've tried to let go of the notion of the story. In fact, now that there are all these different component parts of who I am, there is no conceivable story that can hold it. There are moments that shine with clarity and beauty, and then there are these darker elements that are extremely dark. What am I going to do with them? All I can say is that that's Divine too, and I now have to bring them in and embrace them as who I am, and they're part of me until whenever, until the next stage. ॐ

When I look at my life in a larger sense, the cycles are there – the times where the joy of life is visible, the times when the darkness makes the Light appear invisible, but always the Light is with me, working in its mysterious way.

First published in Issue 13, Life & Death, Spring 2002

marguerite's diary

my first months with cancer

[by Marguerite McAfee]

July 26, 2000

I am not sure I have come to grips yet with the reality of what I am facing – but if I am in denial, then that will be shattered soon. Yesterday I spent four hours at the cancer agency. Anne came and stayed with me. We did *lakita japa* (writing god's name) together and talked about what is going on. It is so good to have spiritual friends who bring me back to reality if I stray.

I have ovarian cancer, and I believe it is in the serious stage, although they have not yet given me exact information. I have the option of joining an international clinical trial, but I have to decide today. I think I will do the trial. It will be more demanding as it includes at least two surgeries and many sessions of chemotherapy, but I would also be given comprehensive treatment and followed closely. And I could give back to the system that is serving me. I will be put in a random group – one group to have surgery first and then chemo, the other group to have chemo first and the surgery twelve weeks after the first treatment. The basic premise of the study is to see if chemo first is a better treatment. Of course, I will have no choice about what course of treatment I will get, but that is where Divine Mother comes in – I will surrender that to her. In fact, it seems I will need to surrender everything to the Divine at this point, my very life. Treatment of one kind or another will begin in the next two weeks.

And I am quite nervous and fearful. Although I am one to stuff my fears down, they are showing up in nightmarish dreams. I had one last night. I'm not sure how to deal with this, but last night I got up and sat and did silent mantra. That helped, and also lying down on the floor beside my Kuanyin. She is so comforting.

I realized that I have been harbouring a silent fear over the months regarding death. A fear that all my family would die and I would be left. How lacking in faith it is for me to think that I would be left alone. I think my recurring dreams about being lost are really about losing my connection with the Divine. That somehow I get into the activities of the day and lose my connection.

And so I am trying to build and strengthen that connection. When I first realized that something was wrong but didn't know what, I moved toward the compassion of Kuanyin. I have been using the Kuanyin oracle book.[1] Her little poems give me courage.

July 27
Reality is coming in closer now. I went again to the cancer agency, this time to ask questions and to sign the consent to be part of the study. I have to undergo further tests to see if I am eligible. I was happy that Anne came with me again because I was nervous. We did *lakita* again and it calmed us both. I am very grateful for her loving friendship. I realize that my nightmare the other night is about my fear and my not acknowledging it. I went to Kuanyin again and help was there. This is the oracle she gave me:

The Right Place
Ascend – it is vital you hole up in the tower,
It's like being in the forest surrounded by thorns…
Heaven's highest wise one decides the fate –
Don't take on things beyond the reach of your powers.

I don't know if I fully understand it all, but the poem tells me to surrender. And so I remembered to offer everything to Kuanyin, even my fear. I hope she doesn't mind my pestering her, because I had to make that offer several times today, and will many times more before Monday when I am scheduled to have another biopsy. I am quite a sissy physically, and have been blessed with a life without a lot of physical pain and so I am quite inexperienced in dealing with it. But deal I must.

It feels like a strange unknown road I am traveling down, not easy, and yet some richness already has emerged – so much love and Light. And humour. Anne and I had a few laughs today amidst the medical milieu.

August 17

It is ten days now since my surgery. Seven days in the hospital – all a little like a dream. A place where there is no choice but to surrender. Under the anesthesia one moment and the next someone saying, "It's all done." No time went by for me, but there were four hours there where other lives were awake and working. How strange time is. There were many nurses changing every twelve-hour shift and then every day or so. It was like Kuanyin, in many forms, coming to my bedside, all through the night, keeping a gentle vigil on my behalf, looking after those vital parts that I was not able to take care of myself. I trusted them and was glad to just surrender to what the moment brought. As I began feeling more awake (I didn't have a lot of pain, but some nausea and headaches for a couple of days), I wanted to go home.

The operation itself was as successful as it could be given the circumstances. This is not a first-stage ovarian cancer I am dealing with but third or fourth, which means it is not confined to the ovaries. A full hysterectomy was done, but the remaining cancer cells need to be dealt with, first with the chemotherapy, and then possibly more surgery. This is how the clinical trial stream which I am part of is planned, but once in the system each case is approached individually. I haven't asked what the prognosis is, but I know my challenge is a big one and I am familiar with the statistics. I really want to stay in the present. For a while I was wondering if I should be planning for living or dying, then realized that we're always in living and dying simultaneously – it's just a little more intense for me at this time. I started rereading the *Tibetan Book of Living and Dying*, by Sogyal

Rinpoche, reading one chapter from the front (Living) and then one from the back (Dying). And so I am trying to rest in the present.

August 18

Yesterday was the first chemotherapy and there will be more to come in three-week intervals. It was a long day. Starting at 7:45 with blood tests, information giving and receiving following that, and then the actual drip, drip of the intravenous potent cocktail for five hours. It was so good to have Anne with me. She did *lakita*, her meditative knitting, spiritual reading, and a little chatting with me from time to time. It is good to have a companion who is not afraid to share this experience with me. I simply lie back in my lounge chair, visualizing the Light permeating my good cells and dissolving those that have become aggressive.

There are two or three others in the room, and at times I am distracted by the conversation that comes and goes as they come and go, all on their own journey. I am the oldest, sixty-seven, and when I see a young, fit-looking twenty-five-year-old man struggling with his diagnosis, I feel compassion for him. How blessed I have been given the tools and the support to follow this journey and learn its lessons. I doze off for an hour and wake refreshed and feeling good. Anne says, "I'm having a good time." And I reply, "Yes, isn't it amazing that you can have a good time in any circumstances – it's all in the mind." When I got home, my sister had drawn back the covers of my bed so I could hop right in. I know the Light was with us all day.

And this morning I feel fine, though not energetic, and on the hospital advice, and my own, am taking quiet time to rest and reflect and write.

August 31

Today I am starting to lose my hair – just two weeks after the first chemo. I thought I might be getting a reprieve (sometimes it doesn't happen until after the second chemo), but yesterday I noticed the top of my head was sensitive and today in the shower my hair was sticking to my face and it was a challenge to get it off and finish my shower without being covered with loose hair. I don't yet know if it will be traumatic for me to lose my hair. I expect to experience some dismay. Hopefully, vanity will lose its grip.

When I last wrote, I had just had chemo and was feeling fine. That lasted only one day. The symptoms moved in, which for me were cramps in the abdomen, nausea, constipation and extreme fatigue. By the second day of this, I wondered if I could handle it. I can't remember the last time I was sick in bed. This lasted a whole week – mostly the fatigue part – and even now, two weeks later, I have very little energy. The next chemo is in a week and so the process repeats itself. They say it's harder each time. I'm not going to speculate on that. I prefer just to have enough information to deal with the present, what is before me now.

I have been well looked after and continue to be grateful for that Divine care. I hope I am open and able to learn the lessens that are inherent in this journey. They may be subtle, though the journey itself is not so subtle.

September 19

Chemo is like dying. This is my second round and I am moving into the living part again, but the first week was very hard, and followed a similar pattern to the first round. The first day is fine, and then for the next three there is dealing with the symptoms – nausea, cramping, headaches, constipation, insomnia – none of them very intense individually, but together, a presence to deal with. Day five, six and seven are about extreme fatigue. I had forgotten that part as I was cutting up a banana for breakfast on day five and had to lie down and rest before I could eat it. This is the dying part – knowing that the energy is not there, not even to hang onto the Light for more than a minute or two, even that I had to surrender. I am so grateful to those who are holding the Light for me. It reminds me of when Papa Ramdas said, "I ask God to hold on to me, because he must know that I cannot hold on to him."

But as the sun shines and my energy comes back, I see I am moving into the living part of this second chemo process. I played my harmonium this morning and will be able to do some practices, reading and who knows what.

September 29 (day of third chemo)

This morning my heart went out to the young woman sitting in the waiting room at the cancer agency. Eight a.m. and I see the telltale tiny round bandage on her arm that indicates that a blood test has been taken, just like mine. But she's too young to have cancer, she can't be more than nineteen and she's sitting there alone. I send her Light – like the Buddhist Tonglen practice – breathing in her pain, along with mine and anyone else's there today, and breathing out Light and healing.

I have moments of feeling weepy today, feeling compassion for those on this journey, and seeing the compassion of the nurses and other personnel as they work with the patients with such patience and care. And I feel grateful for the companionship of Anne again, being there with Light, understanding, acceptance and humour. When I asked Kuanyin what was my message for this round of chemo, it seemed appropriate that the answer was this:

With Love
With love, let a new breeze blow through the house –
The Way is cleared by *Te*, Virtue, as it always was…
So clear your path of the harsh growths that separate you,
When all three can be in harmony, you'll know what's to come.

The oracle felt so right. Love is the basis of all healing, allowing the new to come through. The harsh growth of my body, of my mind – can I embrace them and let them go? What are the three that need to be in harmony? Maybe the body, mind, soul. How do I bring into harmony the dark and the Light? There lies the mystery.

October 15
Thinking back to my third round of chemo… Trudeau died the day before, September 28th. I spent the week watching his memoirs on TV. It was a flashback for me. I lived in Ottawa in 1970 to 1972 when my husband worked for the Liberal party. It was the peak of the Trudeau-mania, and the air was electric with his presence. It was good to watch and pull that part of my life together. I also watched the funeral ceremony and it was very moving – particularly the son's eulogy. And it didn't pass my notice that there I was, in the down part of my chemo, watching the passing of a soul.

Another small insight: I can't have a conscious death without having a conscious life, right up to those last weeks, days, hours, minutes. Not an easy task. When my body is down, I recognize how one can be ready to let the body go, even eager for the release. And when my energy starts coming back, my thoughts go outward. What do I still need to do? I look again at the oracle from that time, its last line, "When all three can be in harmony, you'll know what's to come." I hope so.

How grateful I feel when the energy starts to come back. Energy is so much taken for granted. Not anymore. I have a small window of time between each chemo, which is a treasure. The next round I will be on my own. But I am prepared, I think. My sister Marylin is willing to come over for the few days when I am in intense fatigue. I have a freezer full of food and many offers of more. I am a happy person, because I am starting to understand what Pema Chodron says in the last lines of her book, *When Things Fall Apart*: "This is why it can be said that whatever occurs can be regarded as the path and that all things, not just some things, are workable. This teaching is a fearless proclamation of what's possible for ordinary people like you and me."

November 25

The window of energy is starting to open, so it is a good time for writing. Day eleven, halfway through the fifth chemo. I wake up this morning with an energetic mind full of thoughts of life. A few minutes up and the reality check comes in – my body is way behind my mind and does not have the energy to do the things my mind is suggesting. I am not the body, I am not the mind – but the two are not even together. All the same, I am glad that my mind is lively and not depressed with the struggles of my body.

I asked Kuanyin how I could bring equanimity into this fifth round and her answer was this oracle:

Visible and Invisible
You can't see the moon in its early new days
But isn't it radiant, gold and round, nevertheless?
Wait until mid-month for the Lighting of the Night –
And then its brightness fills the whole circle of the sky.

I can look at my chemo cycle like the cycle of the moon. I don't see the Light in the first half, working with symptoms, yet I know that the Light is always present. And I know that others are holding the trust space for me, holding the

Light. When I pass the mid-point, I know the Light will be more visible, life will begin to have energy again, movement. And the cycle will end, but another will begin. When I look at my life in a larger sense, the cycles are there – the times where the joy of life is visible, the times when the darkness makes the Light appear invisible, but always the Light is with me, working in its mysterious way.

November 29
I have felt my energy recovering more slowly this round and it seems there is a reason. My blood test yesterday showed my hemoglobin count was down and the doctors recommend a blood transfusion. Apparently this is quite common with chemotherapy. And so tomorrow I will go for the transfusion. It will be another long session – maybe six hours – and so another day disappears into the realm of this medical world I am in. Anne, my real live Kuanyin, will accompany me for this session. I cannot express the gratitude I feel for all the Light that is coming my way.

I still don't know if my illness was reflecting a temptation to leave my body, the desire not to be left behind, not to endure the death of family members before my own. Or is the illness about preparation for death, learning to loosen the self-will that is attached to the body and material pleasures, learning to deal with the fears that are attached to death? Or is it surrendering so that I can finish my days in service without the anxieties that can hold me back from giving service freely? I don't really know the answer. And does it really matter that I don't know?

December 11
This is my final chemo, my final ride on the roller coaster. Now I will be moving into a slow steady incline. Dear Kuanyin, please can you guide me through this incline? What will be my focus? My direction?

I feel ready. So many people are waiting in the waiting room for a blood test. I see a beautiful blonde girl about age twenty with her lovely young mother. I do the Tonglen practice for them. I know who the cancer patient is when the young girl gets up to go for her test. My heart goes out to the woman and her child.

My blood test comes soon. This time it didn't hurt and the blood moved easily. I notice two women have chosen, as I have, to wear scarves and hats instead of wigs. I'm happy with the choice. I don't think I would have worn the wig if I had got one. I see a man come in, totally bald, and he looks good. Anne and I wait in the chemo room for the results of the test. We chat and sit quietly and do *lakita*. The nurse brings the okay and we get started about 10:15. It is a good day. The IV goes in easily without discomfort. And the hours pass rather quickly.

An Asian family comes in. Father takes the chair, mother stands by, and daughter is the translator. I think it is their first session. A short daily session for a week for him. It's different for everyone. Later, an older couple comes. This is her first treatment. I can see her anxiety. She takes notes very meticulously as the treatment and side effects are explained. My heart goes out to them.

Later that day…

Wakefulness
Don't rest on your laurels with what you've got;
It's neither "bad," at this time, nor is it "good."
Don't cut a part of yourself off to make a patch;
Don't react like this to make a change…

Kuanyin is telling me to remember to be wakeful. When I am feeling good I have a tendency to slide off the path. Stay on. The first two lines are clear. In fact, I don't know exactly "what I've got." The next moment is unknown, and when it comes, not to be judged by good or bad. I don't know what the next step in this journey is, except that I need to bring wakefulness and equanimity to it. The last two lines are not clear yet, but I have an idea. Do not cut off that part of myself that has integrity and honesty, do not cut off this experience, pretend that it is other than it is. Looking in the mirror and seeing my bald head and sparse eyebrows and eyelashes is a daily reminder that I have been a cancer patient. It is hard to say these words. But to deny or forget this fact would be to discount all the Kuanyins who have come into my life.

There are certain anxieties that go with finishing these six rounds of chemo. First and foremost is that I am not finished; there is a possibility that there could be a need for nine, if the treatment has not completed its job. Or down the road, the cancer will reoccur and will be untreatable. I would prefer that my exit from this life was not cancer. Why? Because I don't yet fully understand why it is my path at this time. I have heart problems and arthritis problems, and I have a better understanding of how they are connected to myself, the Marguerite self. But I think the bottom line about making my exit is that it will happen when I have finished the work that I am able to do in this life. Perhaps the exit route is not that important – or maybe it is. I don't know. ॐ

[UPDATE: Marguerite McAfee died on May 26, 2005, while this book was being produced. One week before her death, she granted us the rights to this article, hoping that it would inspire others having life and death experiences with cancer.]

[1] *Kuan Yin: Myths and Prophecies of the Chinese Goddess of Compassion,* Martin Palmer and Jay Ramsay with Kwok Man-ho (London: Thorsons, 1995).

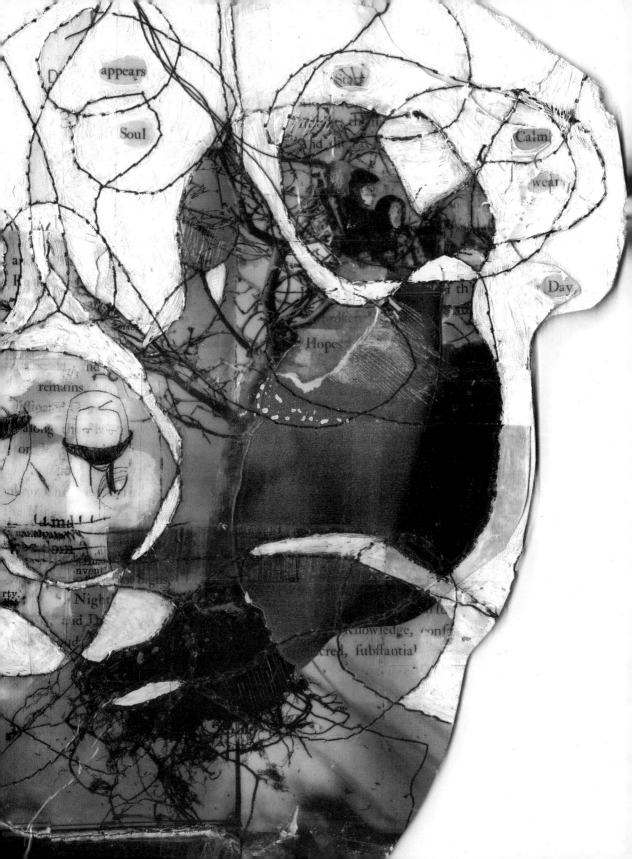

First published in Issue 21, Next Generation, Spring 2004

darkness & light

in the face of violence & violation, how do I keep faith alive?

[by Sikeena Karmali]

Tashkent, Uzbekistan, October 2002

Morning, 8:45 a.m. A phone call: Death in Custody. A taxi driver who gave a lift to two men suspected of being thieves was arrested yesterday. This morning his death was uncovered by family members attempting to visit him in prison. The two robbers were not arrested. The taxi driver died in the police station. He was tortured to death by law enforcement officers. What is unusual about his case is that he has not been alleged to have a connection with any kind of Islamic or other religious activity. Death in custody by torture is routine in Uzbekistan. Freedom of religious worship and expression is not.

Lunchtime. Two Russian human rights activists were arrested for protesting outside the Ministry of Justice. They have been sentenced without trial to forced psychiatric detention. Nobody – friends, relatives, journalists or other activists –

illustration by Cristina Sitja Rubio

is allowed to visit them. One of the women's mothers has managed to sneak into the psychiatric hospital and see her daughter. She took some food for her but not much, as she herself is elderly, ailing and poor. There are rumours based on past such detentions – both women have been detained at least twice in the last two years – that they are being heavily drugged and subjected to severe electric shock therapy. I am trying to pressure the US embassy to convince the Minister of Health and the Minister of Justice to allow me to visit the two women in hospital and inquire about their treatment.

Afternoon. The US embassy. In the hot seat. I am sitting at a long table in a narrow room across from a panel of nine white men in dark suits. Ostensibly we are here to discuss the policies of the US embassy and the human rights program I am attempting to direct. Essentially, they have called this meeting to suss me out. Me: female, young, South Asian, Muslim, non-American, running a program they are financing.

Evening. A journalist, the chief editor of a local government-controlled newspaper, has been sacked for printing a controversial article.

Night. The Che bar. Blaring Eurotechno pop. The daughter of the president of Uzbekistan is gyrating among the elite of Tashkent, in the midst of women whoring themselves to foreign men. The UN Special Raporteur on Torture team, a group of people who blur the distinction between rock star and jet-setting international human rights activist, arrives tonight. We are meeting them here. My tall, dark and handsome friend who blurs that same distinction, between mouthfuls of red Marlboro smoke, tells me about a nineteen-year-old boy in Guantanamo prison camp. He was charged at sixteen years of age for masterminding the "terrorist" bombings in Tashkent on February 19, 1999. One of the bombs almost claimed the president's life. The boy fled to Afghanistan where he was welcomed by the Taliban and became a foot soldier in return for refuge. Now the Uzbeks are asking the Americans to send him back so that they can execute the death penalty of 1999.

Yoga? I have not done a single *asana* in the two months I have been here. Breath? I am not aware that I breathe. Mindfulness? I eat what is put before me – usually fatty lamb and greasy short fat rice. I attempt to pick out the lamb but know that soon I will surrender to it or starve. I have started smoking again. Yes, me, who at home in Montréal eats organic food, who will not put chemicals on her skin or hair, who will wear only clothing made of natural fibres. I am smoking cigarettes. Up to five a day, ten if my nerves are jerking around.

Meditation. My meditation practice consists of a few minutes in the morning, when I am not rushing off to an emergency, or before bed if I have not had a sixteen-hour day and have managed to salvage a few grains of energy for myself. My spiritual practice consists of hot candlelit baths with rose essence and silent chanting of my *zikr* in the midst of whatever I happen to be doing when I feel as if my mind might explode. Peace? Where? Nonviolence? How?

Darkness. I am surrounded by empty politicians. Bigwig names with heavyweight titles, representatives of international organizations and powerful Western governments. Working for peace, for stability and security. A cacophony of deceit. The lechery of pompous stuffy diplomats. How will I find the Light again?

Human rights defenders from all over Uzbekistan travel days by bus and car, even on foot, to come to our office in the capital. They smell of dust and un-washing, effusing the unpleasant breath of malnutrition and rotting teeth. These men and women have risked their lives, risked the very freedom to walk and talk, to breathe, simply by coming here, to my office to speak with me or my staff. Most of them we will turn away. Unable to help. Telling them the same story they have heard a hundred times.

How do we survive injustice? What is the correct posture for that? Which breath shall I breathe through this? How can I confront violations of the most basic human rights, torture, the taking of life, and still move forward? Most of my colleagues, that is the expatriates here, drown themselves in drink or numb themselves with vacant sex. In some cases, both. One seems to lead to the other.

Surrender. I have surrendered to the darkness, although I cannot see what lies before me. My days are spent in a storm of wild chaos. I shuttle between the Uzbek authorities; the bickering politics of local human rights defenders who are constantly trying to outdo each other to attract international attention and favour; and the victims of human rights violations whom my mandate dictates that I should ignore. International organizations and embassies who pay long-faced lip service to the need to do something about the outrageous human rights situation in the country are constantly phoning to arrange meetings, talks, coffees and lunches with their high-profile, $1000-a-day "expert" consultants. Sneaky journalists hover around firing algebraic questions of politics and diplomacy, hoping to catch and expose the Americans at their tripartite dirty game of foreign aid in return for a military base from which to wage the war on Afghanistan, while funding my human rights program to acquiesce the international community. Lastly, there is the SNB – the new Uzbek version of the KGB. In addition to bugging all my phones and my computer, they keep two cars parked outside my house, two more outside my office and follow me around, everywhere.

When I walk in the woods and come upon a darkened passage, I don't crumble to the ground and lie there. I don't stop to savour the darkness. I don't question the night, fighting it, hollering for the day to come back. No, I accept it and move on. In my work, just as in the woods, I keep walking, knowing that the darkness will end. Unable to see, unable to even imagine the next moment, I walk on. Mindfulness? No. I am taking in neither the big picture nor the details. I can see neither. Am not even contemplating my intention. Just putting one foot before the other and moving forward. One breath at a time. Knowing that the Light will come. Believing it.

The world is not just. I know that. I have always known that. However acute my pained sense of justice, no matter how hard I fight, there will always be injustice. I cannot change that. Some things we just have to accept. The world is not fair, but God is. So I have surrendered the justice of those for whom I can do nothing, to God. I pray for them. I pray that God will be merciful toward them. I pray for their strength, that they may come to resolution and thereby to absolution. I pray that they shall be free from this, that they too will walk through the darkness and come into Light.

Lost in the turmoil of my darkness, shadowed by it, I do not see when power struggles in Washington or when the situation inside the very program I direct becomes unjust. How far do you surrender? When does blindness come? When do you take a stand? At which moment do you fight the darkness? Knowing. Knowing full well that you will probably lose.

What is there to gain in fighting that which you cannot control? Nothing, really. Nothing you can measure or count. Nothing that I can list here to convince you. Only a lightness of the breath. A clarity of the eye. Spiritual beauty. Grace. A luminescence devoid of cosmetic artistry.

Light. It is my faith that brings the Light. Nothing more. Nothing less. We are at yet another international conference. Political muscle backed by pockets bulging with economic promise. All the big players are here. What I didn't know is that my Imam, my spiritual guide, His Highness the Aga Khan, is also here. He is a famous man, delivering an important lecture. He is not accessible, in the manner that the Dalai Lama and the Pope are not accessible.

I attend the lecture. When it ends I am struggling through a thick crowd to find my staff. But he finds me. My Imam finds me in the midst of an airless crowd. He is ensconced by aggressive journalists, microphones jutting out surrounding his face like diamonds setting off a jewel. Photographers are snapping away. He stands back, ignoring them to speak to me. We have a conversation during which I try to mask the fact that my knees are shaking. My Imam has come to Tashkent, Uzbekistan to bless me. I sent the East/West issue of *ascent* to his secretariat last autumn, which included an article I had written. I know that the question of East and West is close to his heart. He wants one world. He asks about my life. What I will do next. I speak to him mechanically, not registering the conversation until much later. What I see is his shining eyes and beaming smile. I know now why I came to Uzbekistan.

Montréal, Canada, October 2003

Home. Here I am, one year later. I am in Montréal again. Hoping to live a more ordinary life. Trying to push away the dramatics of hopping continents. Avoiding looking evil in the eye. I dream of a stable life, knowing that it will never be. That stillness which I crave is transitory. It does not last. When it does, life becomes death. Living is a dynamic activity. It is about moving, shifting, learning, growing. Opening to your fate. Be-ing.

I have wounds to heal. The Light shall heal them. Without darkness, the Light is less dazzling. Coming through pain, love will stun you. Surviving your suffering will unleash your strength. I understand this now.

I miss Tashkent. I miss Umida, Luba and Dilmurad.
I miss the smell of my house.
I miss my garden.
I miss the walk to the Caravan and those crazy Russian salads.

I miss the hot naan that Dilmurad would scorch his hands on to bring to me.
I miss Umida's unshakeable strength and Hayot's dumbfounded silences.
I miss quirky Raykhan and the cake lady.
I miss the love of our small office before you came.

I do not miss the anguish sweeping through the streets.
I do not miss the hollow sockets of shame.
I do not miss the cutting dismissals of bureaucracy.
I do not miss the conspiring whispers of secret fears.

I do not miss the coffees at the Boumi – my desperate attempt to inject routine
        normalcy into the day.
I do not miss the harlots at the Che Bar, as in Che Guevara.
I do not miss the numbing cold of my unheated office.
I do not miss the susurrus of lies and naked libido of pink, bloated men at
        diplomatic receptions.

I miss Luba, in the mornings, imploring me to stay in bed and not go to work.
I miss the light at dusk on the pomegranate tree.
I miss the honey made of wood flowers and the green tea with lemon.
I miss my family of Uzbek colleagues whose courage I cannot name.

    It is they, not the Americans, not my office in Washington and certainly
not the embassy social circuit, who helped me survive when I was alone. Before
you came. ॐ

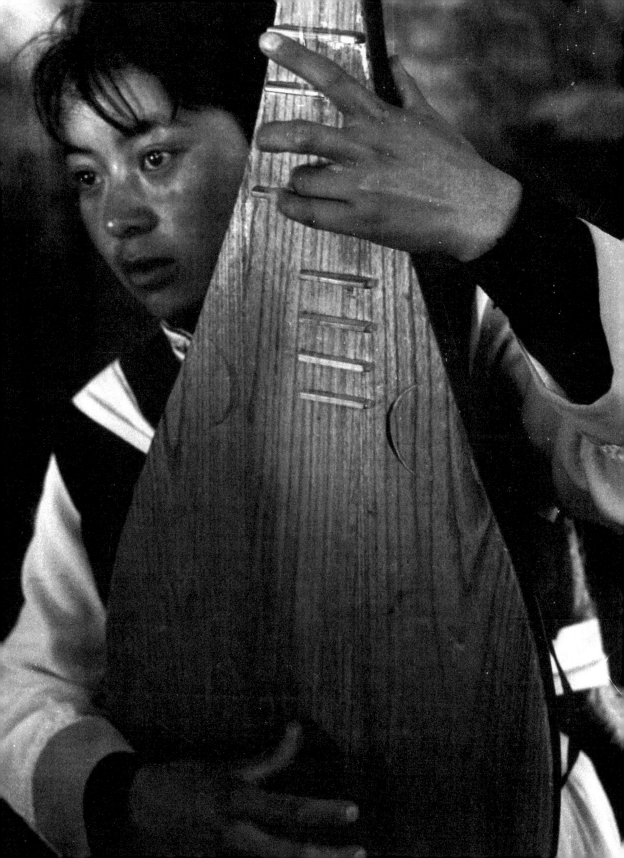

First published in Issue 14, Sound, Summer 2002

17 hours in china
where is guan yin?

[by Sarah E. Truman]

the bus is overcrowded. On the road, travelers with big bags try to flag us down, but there is no room for them. We reached full capacity a long time ago. People are standing everywhere in the aisles. Food, suitcases and fireworks in colourful packages spill out of the overhead racks. The air is thick and hot and smoky. Almost everyone on the bus is smoking. The men standing in the aisle smoke while hanging on to the backs of seats, the driver smokes while he grinds the gears and honks the horn, and beside the driver, seated on the big old-fashioned hump of an engine, four men in grey-black suits sit smoking.

I can't open the window because the woman in front of me is vomiting. She has been vomiting off and on for about an hour. The woman in front of her is also vomiting. In fact, there are six people vomiting on the bus. Everyone on the bus is either vomiting or smoking.

I'm getting used to scenes like this. I've been in China for six months, working in Nanjing. Nanjing is in central east China, near Shanghai. This is my

photo by Sarah E. Truman

first holiday. I wanted to visit southern China, so I decided to come to Yunnan Province, which borders Myanmar, Vietnam and Tibet.

Northern Yunnan is populated by Naxi, descendants of Tibetan nomads who migrated here hundreds of years ago. Out the window, I see green fields and hills and mountains in the distance. Houses – little white houses with innumerable identical black-tiled roofs – peek out in every direction. People in colourful clothing, traditional Naxi clothing, are walking, working and carrying in the fields. The Naxi have managed to maintain their customs, dialect and even their own pictorial language through the turmoil of the past few decades in China. The next few decades will likely bring another challenge to their customs with a steady stream of tourists entering the region, both foreigners and the new Chinese middle class.

"I understand nothing of this."

Razvan is awake. "It's like a different language. I understand nothing," he says.

Razvan is a herbalist from Romania. He has lived in China for five years studying Chinese herbs and speaks fluent Putonghua (standard Chinese Mandarin). I met Razvan last autumn in the garden below my apartment in Nanjing. I had just bought a new kite and was keen on flying it. As I walked past him he saw the kite and told me it wouldn't work because the wind was too soft. Instead of flying the kite, we got into a small argument about wind and became friends.

"You know, the further you get from Beijing, the more you hear a different language altogether."

I nod at him with superficial understanding. I don't know enough standard Chinese to make any sweeping comparisons, but what I do know sounds very different from what I am hearing.

The tape just flipped over again, the same tape of Chinese pop songs that we've listened to since we got on the bus at noon. There are five songs on each side. I'm not sure what the lyrics are about but I think they talk of love. Very dramatic. The woman behind me knows most of the songs, but she sometimes has trouble holding the key. A man in the aisle is singing as well, another song altogether. He sings the same line over and over again in between drags of his cigarette.

"Why is he singing on top of the radio? And why does he keep saying the same thing over and over?" I ask aloud, not expecting an answer. I'm becoming irritable and fidgety, and my legs are sore from sitting in these little seats.

I close my eyes and think of the temple I visited this morning before I got on the bus. I arrived early and found the place overrun by tourists. The temple was typically Chinese, in that it came complete with entrance fees, glossy tickets with misleading photos of statues, cameras everywhere and tawdry religious junk for sale. I've visited many temples in China and discovered, to my dismay, that a lot of them are nothing more than false-fronted amusement parks kept up as money-makers.

I felt embarrassed this morning. Embarrassed for China, for religion and for myself being part of the façade. I vowed to never visit a religious site again, when a service began. To my surprise several seeming tourists were actually lay practitioners. They slipped dark brown robes over their street clothes and were suddenly perched in front of prayer pillows. I've heard rumours of people being paid to perform religious services and I almost accused them of doing so, but then I listened.

They were chanting to the bodhisattva Guan Yin [Kuanyin], and they were chanting with heart. I could hear it once I let myself listen. It sounded sweet and sincere. I knew the mantra so I joined in. The woman who was in charge of closing the doors allowed me to stay in the temple during the service. Maybe because I was singing, too.

It is difficult to understand the coexistence of religion and Communism, but they seem to coexist, at least superficially, here in China. Although the past fifty years here have seen some serious damage to Chinese spirituality, there seems to be at least a feigned tolerance for religious sites, with newly rebuilt temples, churches and mosques. The government certainly has a monetary interest in religious practice, and it often feels that tourism is the only reason temples are rebuilt and kept up. Maybe Communism and religion have found a middle ground – commerce. Still, I've heard that the CCP does not allow nonatheists to become party members.

"Nan wu guan shi yin pu sa."

"Now you're singing on top of the music," Razvan says to me.

I look at Razvan and smile. The man in the aisle is still singing but I don't mind it so much. We're heading to a small city with a large Naxi population where Razvan's wife, Christina, studies Chinese music with a private teacher. It's the eve of Spring Festival and Christina has arranged some celebratory activities for us. Tomorrow I want to borrow Christina's bike and visit an old monastery complex outside town. I have a particular interest in the place because of the name of one of its temples: Xia Guan Yin Si.

I have a long-time affection for Guan Yin, the compassionate *bodhisattva* who promises to deliver all beings from suffering. In the teachings, she's said to live in the south sea on an island near the purple bamboo grove and cave of tidal sound. One of the major reasons I came to China was to see what's happened to her and her places of worship in the past half-century.

Since arriving I've encountered a myriad of Guan Yins: Guan Yin flashing red light dangly things hanging from the rear-view mirror in taxis, Guan Yins in water that if you shake them upside down will be showered in little plastic coins symbolizing wealth, Guan Yin stickers in gum machines. At first I thought that kitsch and rebuilt statues were what Guan Yin has been reduced to here in modern China. But it's said that Guan Yin will manifest in any form, whatever expediency suggests to help devotees – so maybe the modern mind likes trinkets. Or maybe all I see is trinkets, and I'm missing the point. It's difficult to be objective about something as subtle and subjective as Guan Yin. Still, I'm looking for traces of her and her devotees here, trying to get a sense of her presence in modern China. I don't know exactly what I'm looking for, or when I'll know that I've found it. But I'm still searching.

I think we're getting close to our destination because the bus has come alive with another kind of racket – cellular phones. An amazing number of Chinese carry one. They have a way of yelling into the phones that makes me a little uncomfortable. I associate yelling with anger or miscommunication and imagine that they are fighting when they're merely having a conversation about where to meet for dinner. Almost everyone on the bus is on the phone now and shuffling to arrange their bags.

Christina is waiting for us at the station, waving and hopping.

"You are late. We missed dinner at the guest house," she says as we arrange our bags. We apologize and she tells us we'll have to drop off our bags at the guest house and we can eat along the way to meet up with some of her friends.

The restaurant is full. We manage to squeeze three short chairs and a table onto the platform sitting directly below the grey garage entrance door. The restaurant is like so many in China, each with its own grey garage door and short tables. The walls are white and wet and decorated with pictures advertising foods that are obviously not on the menu. I sit facing a large glossy photo of two crystal glasses, some candies, a pile of apples, German chocolates strewn across the foreground, and two hotdogs sliced onto an open-faced melted cheese sandwich. I've seen many photographs of this genre since I arrived in China. Maybe they like the colours.

Beside the photo, in the corner, with two red candles and some fruit, sits a grubby white porcelain Guan Yin, silently observing the dining.

"What do you want to eat?" asks Christina. She has long, soft hands that always seem to be moving as if they have a mind of their own. Musician's hands. We agree on some standard dishes: fried sliced potatoes and green peppers (*Qing Jiao Tu Dou Si*), spicy family-style tofu (*Jia Chang Dou Fu*), four-season green beans with garlic (*Si Jie Dou*), rice and tea.

"That man wearing glasses is from Beijing," says Razvan. Christina agrees. "You can understand him?" I ask. They nod.

The man from Beijing has thick squarish glasses and the Chairman Mao hairstyle that some older Chinese men sport. He and his friends all wear Western suits and black leather dress shoes. When I first came to China I thought that every man was a businessman because they all wear suits and dress shoes. Then I began to notice that people wore suits regardless of what they were doing. They wear suits to dig ditches, suits to garden, suits to drive the bus. Not the expected Mao Zedong blue-grey revolutionary suits, but 1980s shoulder-padded business suits.

The man from Beijing is making a toast, *ganbei,* which means dry glass. He notices us noticing him and says *lao wai* to his friends. *Lao wai* means foreigner. The whole table turns toward us, smiling. They fill their glasses and come over to our table for a toast. We stand and take part. The man from Beijing and his friends empty the glass. I sip and grimace. *Bai jiu* is a popular drink made from rice – 52 percent alcohol and tastes like it.

When the men learn that Christina and Razvan speak Chinese, we are invited to dine with them. The table is a sea of familiar dishes, fishes and soups. Razvan and the man from Beijing discuss something; Christina chats with another man. The others try to include me and we go through all the "Where are you from? How long have you been in China? Why are you a vegetarian?" and exhaust my Chinese. Then they let me be, occasionally placing a piece of food on my plate, telling me that fish *bu shi rou* (is not meat).

"Do you understand any of this?" Christina asks.

"I understand a word or two here and there, but don't worry, I'll just listen," I say, and I listen.

When I first came to China, the language was a wall of sound. I could sit in a restaurant like this and hear nothing but noise – rising and falling sounds like a song, staccato but slurred language. Wholly unintelligible. I used to catch myself trying to fit sounds I heard into English words or sounds. This got me nowhere.

There is a man who sells newspapers in the alley beside my apartment. Every day at exactly 3:20 he comes and calls out the name of the paper. I couldn't understand what he was saying. *A guava ball* is what I heard for about three months. Then one day I decided to investigate. I took my Chinese friend and we waited in the alley until the paper man came. It turned out that the name of the paper is *Yangtze Wan Bao*. My friend admitted that the man was slurring, but insisted that the man was in fact saying *Yangtze Wan Bao*.

After that incident I decided to give up listening to words for awhile and tried a new strategy: listening to the spaces between words, the silence where words end. I became an expert in spaces.

But lately Chinese words have begun to fill the silence. The wall of sound is coming apart brick by brick and I catch words here and there. The silence is more difficult to hear. I look at the Guan Yin in the corner. Her name, "Guan Shi Yin," literally translates as "observe world sound." I wonder if she listens to the silence or just the sounds.

Xiao jie xiao jie! The man beside me is calling me little-big sister. He wants to toast to spring. I have another small sip of the *bai jiu*. I still have over half a glass in front of me. I look at Razvan and without taking my eyes off his, pick up the glass and pour the remainder into my rice bowl. A friend taught me that if you look casual while you dump out *bai jiu* no one notices. Maybe everyone is secretly dumping out their *bai jiu*.

We're in the old town, racing to meet Miss Liu, Christina's music teacher, and some of Miss Liu's friends at a concert. The streets are granite and there are little canals and bridges everywhere. All the tourist shops are alight and busy with shoppers. I can hear the prelude of fireworks coming from courtyards of all the identical white houses as we hurry through the maze of narrow streets.

The theatre is oversold, but Christina has tickets. Miss Liu and her friends have reserved seats for us on the balcony. At least fifty people are without seats, standing in little pockets and corners and behind poles all over the theatre. Everyone is smoking and eating and cellular phones are ringing while the musicians tune their ancient instruments. I'm sitting between Miss Liu and Christina.

"See the man with the blue shirt? That man is Miss Liu's uncle." Christina whispers in my left ear. "He is seventy-two years old and famous in town for his erhu playing. He's lived here since he was young. He taught Miss Liu and her sister, but only Miss Liu still plays; she is carrying on the tradition."

Miss Liu looks anything but traditional. She smokes Marlboro cigarettes and has dyed reddish hair and a tight red shirt with a huge butterfly collar. And she's wearing tinted glasses in a dark theatre. Miss Liu looks more like a pop star than an erhu player. We've hardly spoken, but I like Miss Liu already.

The orchestra begins with a song about spring. The instruments twang, wiggle and bend the notes almost out of tune, but the musicians hold it together. The sound is hopeful but somehow sad.

"Do you like?" Miss Liu whispers in my right ear after the first song.

"Yes, but it always sounds a little sad to me."

"It is sad. Look how old they are," she says and then pauses. "And there's not very many young people interested in learning. Even out of my family, I am the only one that continues and we are Han, not Naxi. The Naxi people are losing their tradition in music. You are lucky to hear some of these songs and these musicians." She lets out a white cloud of smoke.

I look at the orchestra again. The majority of the members are over sixty and there are a few who must be over eighty. Even their instruments are old, blackened. There's two youngish women in the group, each playing a zither. The music sounds even more melancholy to me now, like the memory of something lost, something I can't remember.

Outside the theatre the festivities are in full swing. We walk out into mayhem. Children run everywhere with lighters in one hand and cherry bombs in the other. Sparklers, piles of paper money burn all over the street. Incense and laughter.

"Spring Festival was once a time that everyone went home and the shops were closed, but look at this. Everything open. It's almost midnight!" Razvan says with a big smile as he stops to examine a bronze bell.

"What? Are you going to shop now?" Christina says, irritated with him.

"I can't look?"

"You never just look. You always buy. This from the Qing Dynasty, that from the Song Dynasty, this from the Ming Dynasty," Christina imitates him in an official-sounding voice.

I love it when non-native speakers speak English to each other for my benefit; it's like a play. I leave them arguing in the brightly lit bell shop and run to catch up with Miss Liu.

"We must hurry to the main street for the fireworks," Miss Liu says as she hands me a bottle of plum liquor. I take a swig. It tastes nice but burns my throat. I take another swig. Miss Liu and her friends have bought some fireworks. Little red balls of gunpowder that explode when they hit something hard. They're throwing them at each other's feet and laughing. It seems like a dangerous game on such narrow stone streets. And so loud. Miss Liu hands me some little red balls. I whip them at a wall. The noise is different when I make it.

The main street looks like a war zone. Grey smoke clouds around the street lights and red scraps of paper and ashes blowing in the breeze. Children not old enough to feed themselves stand holding miniature cannons aimed at the street blasting colours and noise. Men on big tricycles, who by day might sell vegetables, ride up the street selling piles of fireworks. Then we come to the grey garage doors, about ten of them, filled with fireworks. There must be thirty people in each store, all sorting, bargaining and buying.

"It's midnight," Miss Liu announces, first in Chinese, then in English. And it begins. People line the street. Some carry garbage bags full of fireworks. They are mainly men, several with eye patches, cigarettes in one hand and every possible combination of fireworks in the other, blasting blasting blasting them into the night. Some make pretty colours against the nuclear sky, but mainly they're noisemakers, ground-shakers. I stand in a corner, my ears plugged, listening for a moment of silence.

Miss Liu's house is an old house, identical to all the others in the old town from the outside. It was her father's house. There's a main gate opening onto a courtyard. One red lantern hangs from the tree above the garden and two hang from the balcony above the porch. Two men play Chinese chess in the yard with two women. I can hear music coming from the room between the red lanterns. Miss Liu leads me to the music.

In the sparsely furnished room with hardwood floors and a high ceiling, several musicians sit, doing what can only be described as jamming. Although I recognize most of them from the fireworks, Miss Liu introduces them as her "bohemian friends." There's one erhu, one Gu Qing, a flute and I don't know the names of the other pretty instruments.

"And this is my boyfriend Phil. Phil's his English name, he speaks English." She flops down beside a man on the couch. "Phil was born in Northern Yunnan, he's a painter." I sit with Phil while Miss Liu and her friends play.

"You don't play?" I ask Phil.

"No, I just listen. I paint, and I like to know that someone might look at what I make. So when my friends play music, I try to listen."

And we listen.

"You should join the orchestra," I say to Miss Liu's band after a time.

"Maybe some day, but they're much better than we," Miss Liu responds.

"Yeah, they were good, and old. Even their instruments are old and blackened," I say. Everyone is quiet. Miss Liu looks at the wok on the floor that holds embers of a fire instead of food.

"Their instruments are black because they were buried," Miss Liu says.

And I understand. During the Cultural Revolution many musicians buried their instruments in the fields and the woods to protect themselves. It was dangerous to be a music maker. The music literally went underground. I look at the musicians and wonder what they've seen in their lives, what their parents have seen.

I think of how the instruments had to be buried, but they couldn't kill the music. The music keeps changing; it can't be forced to stay a certain way. Like everything else, it's evolving. Miss Liu and her bohemian friends might be the future of the old-style music.

"Let's have some noodles," Miss Liu suggests. Everyone shuffles outside to the table between the two red lanterns. The chess players have gone. It must be almost four in the morning, and I'm losing confidence in making it back to the guest house before dawn. We sit around the table with blankets on our knees, the wok with embers warms our legs. Phil arrives with candles that throw shadows on the garden. Miss Liu arrives with steaming noodles and we eat.

"What is on the red cord around your neck?" Miss Liu asks me as she chews her noodles.

"It's an Indian symbol called Lalita. It's the point from which the universe emanates."

"Oh, I thought it was a Chinese sign. We wear jade on red thread around our necks for protection." She pulls out a little jade Guan Yin to show me.

"Guan Yin!"

"You know?" she asks.

"Yes."

"We believe that if you wear jade and you fall, the jade may break but you will not be hurt," says Phil.

"And why Guan Yin?" I ask.

"Because."

I'm reminded of the Guan Yin temple, the purpose in my coming to town. I excuse myself as everyone lights their cigarettes. I have to get to bed so I don't sleep all day tomorrow. I want to see the temple in the morning.

Miss Liu and Phil want to walk me back to the guest house but I know I'm close. They walk me to the gate and point me in the right direction. The streets are quiet except for the occasional firecracker and the river running constant in its stone gully. There is no moon and no hint of dawn.

Beside the guest house is a public toilet. It's open all night because few people in the area have private toilets. A woman sits in the room between the Gents' and Ladies' toilets. Her job is to collect two Mao from every customer, night and day. She has a dim light in there, a narrow bed and a scratchy radio. I recognize the music playing on the radio! It sounds very familiar but I can't place it. I stand near the window out of her view and listen. I hear the pattern of the song but I can't hear the tune. It's like I'm listening wrong. I'm listening to the spaces between the song instead of the melody. I only hear a gentle wah wah wah.

Quickly, as though someone turned the song around and began to play it properly, I can hear it, clear as day.

"Wild horses couldn't drag me away...Wild wild horses..." The Stones. It seems awfully out of place. I'm confident that the woman in the toilet speaks no English. Maybe she listens to the silence instead of the sounds.

The sky is bluing as I lie down to sleep. I can hear firecrackers in the distance and roosters are crowing.

Christina and Razvan stand at the foot of my bed.

"Are you awake?"

"I am now."

"Sorry, we were worried when we lost you last night. Did you stay with Miss Liu?"

"Yeah. What time is it?"

"Almost eight. They're having breakfast and firecrackers in a minute."

And the firecrackers begin, just outside the courtyard, unbelievably loud. I have no chance of sleeping here. Razvan and Christina are both sitting on the bed asking me questions about last night and whether I'm still going to the temple or if I'd like to go shopping instead. The firecrackers are blasting and everyone in the guest house seems to be yelling. I resign myself to get up and go to the temple. I borrow Christina's bike and bow out of breakfast.

I feel like I'm riding away from a bombing. All through the streets the children throw firecrackers and those little balls of gunpowder. No one else seems to notice the explosions. Women wash clothes in the river and sweep and carry everything from fowl to small children in wicker baskets on their backs. Men sit along the road, smoking, selling breakfast. I come to wider streets and traffic. I join the bikes and head west out of town with my shadow in front of me.

One of the nicest things in the south is bamboo. Strong and green and whispering everywhere. The temple is set in bamboo, at the base of a hill. It looks like most temples I've visited: tall yellow walls, black-tiled roofs, a new gate that was likely rebuilt because the first one was "damaged by fire" during the Cultural Revolution. It's awful how many temples were destroyed during those years. And sometimes it wasn't the temples that were ruined, just the statues, a hand broken here, a face smashed there. One of the most destructive acts I've seen evidence of was a fresco of a *bodhisattva*. The whole thing was intact except the eyes – they were dug out round and blank. Something about that image haunts me; it was too precise.

Several makeshift booths stand in front of the gate selling statues and pictures and incense. The vendors all call to me, saying, "Looky, looky," and waving little *maitrayas* and plastic *malas*. Again, I have mixed feelings about my contribution to the commercialized tourism of religious sites here in China. Is this what religion evolves into? I wonder what I support in being here. A new, more insidious destruction? I don't know. I pay my entrance fee and enter the large courtyard where some visitors chat, pose for photos and burn huge sticks of incense.

There are several halls in different directions off the courtyard. I enter the one to my left. It's filled with Arhats. Three storeys of Arhats line the walls, staring, laughing, google-eyed and looking very unhuman. They scare me a little. I wonder if that's the point. I can hear my heart beating in my ears.

A round-faced monk in a mustard suit sits at a small desk in the corner. "*Nin hao*," he says with a big toothy smile.

"*Guan Yin Si zai nar?*" I ask. He stares at me a little, and then directs me out the door and across the courtyard toward a gate.

A little sign, in Chinese characters, reads *Xia Guan Yin Si* (Lower Guan Yin Temple). The sign points through the woods and up the hill. I pass through the gate, excited to visit Guan Yin's own temple. Somewhere that she can sit and observe the world's sounds without distraction.

I'm at the top of the green hill. There's no one around. I approach the temple. I can read the name *Xia Guan Yin Si* written in Chinese characters above the three identical doors that stand open. But it looks empty. I can see through to the other side where three other doors stand wide open.

I feel dizzy.

My flesh tingles as I approach the temple. It's bare. Dirt floor. Nothing on the walls, no altar, no lights. No Guan Yin.

Nothing. Completely empty.

A woman in a blue shirt appears from nowhere. "*Mei you Guan Yin*," she says and spits on the floor.

I walk out the back door and cry a little because it's so perfect. The whole thing is perfect.

The woman is following me and speaking, but I don't understand what she's saying. I smile sadly and she walks away.

I'm alone, listening to the wind in the bamboo behind the empty Guan Yin temple. I know what it means. I don't know what it means. ॐ

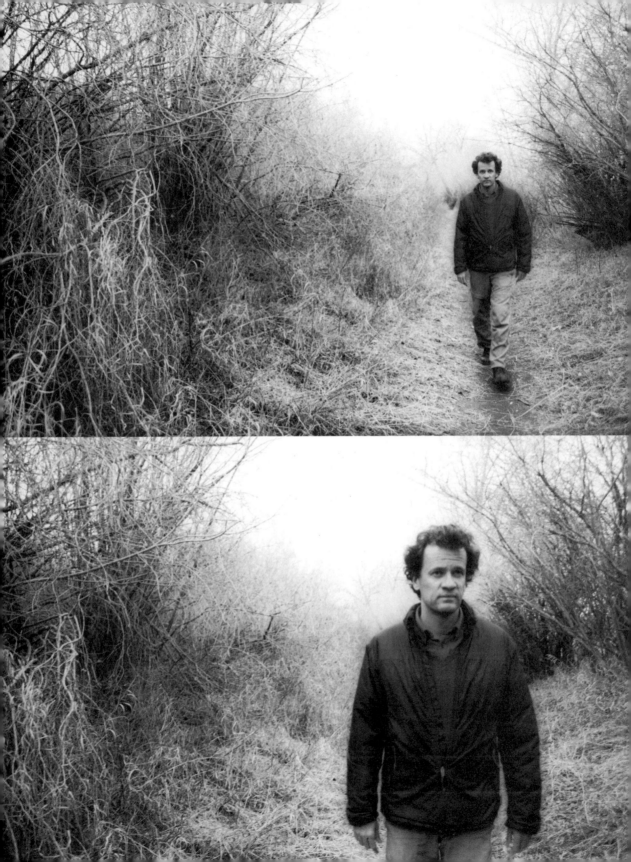

First published in Issue 22, Travel, Summer 2004

adrift with yann martel

the author of *life of pi* asks how to be more profoundly human

[Yann Martel interviewed by Bruce McCoubrey]

●

in a sense," Yann Martel says, "I started traveling before I was even born." Born in Spain, the son of Canadian diplomat parents, Yann got a taste of the adventure in travel early on, and is no stranger to remarkable journeys. He is the highly acclaimed author of *Life of Pi*, winner of the coveted Man Booker Prize in 2002. The hero of the book, Pi Patel, finds himself cast adrift on the Pacific Ocean with a 450-pound Royal Bengal tiger called Richard Parker. With this as the scene, Yann unravels a story of survival and faith that will "make you believe in God," as one character says.

Yann's own exploration of faith began while studying philosophy at Trent University. Yann found the academic environment unappealing and realized that he was looking for something "more holistic, more experiential." It was about this time that he discovered yoga, a discovery that was to prove pivotal to his exploration of the spiritual life. Once a self-professed religious cynic, Yann began to transform himself into someone whose faith is now an integral part of his worldview.

photo by Frances Robson

In fact, questions of faith and of how to live life to its fullest have been the driving force behind his yoga practice, his journeys around the globe and his writing life.

Through his explorations of belief, survival and, in his forthcoming book, the human response to evil, Yann has proven that he is a writer and individual who is not afraid to cast himself adrift with the really tough questions, both personal and universal, and land somewhere unexpected.

ascent caught up with him at the Saskatoon Public Library where he is a writer-in-residence. Now temporarily settled on the prairies, Yann relies on his imagination and his research to take him to faraway places.

Bruce McCoubrey   You recently spent five months as a visiting lecturer at the Free University of Berlin teaching on "The Animal in Literature." You were also researching your next book. Tell us about the premise and your hopes for the book.

Yann Martel   In *Life of Pi,* I was interested in looking at matters of faith and spirit. In the next one, I want to look at great evil. Not so much how do we live with great evil that is in front of us, but how do we live with it afterwards. Once we have lived a trauma, how do we speak of it, how do we remember it, with what words, and how do we come to live with it? It's easy to live with goodness. If I win a million dollars, I can live with that. I have had a good meal and I can live with that. But how do you live with ingratitude, how do you live with lies, how do you live with violence, how do you live with homicide? That destroys in people, in most normal people, the capacity to move forward. So this next book is very different from *Life of Pi.* It's a fable using a monkey and a donkey that takes place on an enormous shirt. It's going to be a fable on the Shoa, the Holocaust. These animals will be asking themselves how do we live with the horror. I am not interested in doing a documentary book on the Holocaust. There is all the information one needs out there. I am interested in the next step. The books that I write, I write because I am trying to understand something, explore something – not necessarily to come to an answer – but to at least understand the questions that should be asked.

BM   You have said that the main theme of Life of Pi *is: "Life is a story. You can choose your story. And a story with an imaginative overlay is the better story." What for you has been the better story?*

YM   The better story for me is one in which this material world – this world that is so present, that seems so un-illusory – is supported by another world that makes sense of it. For me, the better story is that somehow, in a way I don't understand, evil makes sense.

I said "imaginative overlay" because I was hesitant of using the word "religious" or "spiritual." But the first step in a religious pilgrimage is an acknowledgement that we cannot understand everything. Our ego's understanding is finite.

The question is, can we let go of this scientific obsession to find out the reason for everything, find out the causality of everything? Some things do not have a cause that we can understand and that is all right. Is it possible to have faith and then use reason to help you understand your faith and what you can do with your faith?

BM   One of the ideas I took away from Life of Pi *was that faith and the will to live fully are inextricably linked. Have these elements come together in your own life?*

YM   I have always yearned for that to happen, but the problem with yearning to live fully in a world that is strictly materialist is that you cannot find it. Reason itself delivers no reason to be alive, delivers no reason to use reason. Reason is a wonderfully powerful tool, intoxicating in its own way, but it doesn't tell you why you are alive. It doesn't go deeper.

In a strictly materialist context, it is very hard to live fully, as living fully would be viewed in terms of material things. We live in a material world and we cannot deny we are material creatures and we need material comforts. But this weighing of kilograms of material goods is not the way to reach a full life. So for years I lived in an agnostic way.

I think people who are seeking some sort of sense of ultimate meaning in a material context substitute religious ideologies with secular ones. Take ecology, for example – some people who are involved in the environmental movement, their vision of reality, of nature, is quasi-religious. They talk about nature being sacred, which is just not a term that makes any sense when you are a zoologist looking at animals. There is nothing sacred about the way a tiger behaves in India.

People are searching for something that goes beyond the material, but it is very difficult to do that if you are suspicious of any spiritual questioning. What happened in my life was that I was seeking meaning in a materialistic context and couldn't find one. So finally I said, why don't I have a look at religion, defining the word very broadly, and see what that yields.

BM Prior to writing Life of Pi, *you described yourself as a religious cynic. It was through the research for that book that you started to embrace a worldview that has given root to your own faith. Describe your journey to arrive at that point. Was yoga a central element of that journey or was it something altogether different?*

YM Yoga was definitely something that helped me.

When you are doing *Savasana,* when you are breathing in and you're relaxing – that is the best way to let yourself imagine that maybe there is something other than the material. So that gentle loosening up, loosening up, loosening up, starting with the body, did predispose me to question religion in a more sympathetic light when I went to India.

Another element of that journey was simply reading, informing myself. One of the first steps in any kind of religious traveling is acknowledging that there is something greater than us. Part of that acknowledgement is accepting that you can't know everything and therefore you must learn. A wonderful way to learn is through reading, so I began reading some sacred texts – the Bible, the Koran, the Bhagavad Gita, the Upanishads.

I also was witness to the spiritual practices of others, the real spiritual practice of others. I know two Catholic priests in Montréal who truly live in the spirit of Christ. And in India, I saw *sadhus,* people on pilgrimages, people living a spiritual life in a concrete way.

I know this is bastardizing a quote from William James, but "a man will often take as true something that will make him feel better." One of the things that helped me take this spiritual stuff seriously was that involving myself with it, in it, made me feel better, made me feel more connected, made me feel more profoundly human. Therefore I took it to be something significant, something true. So the effect on me made me continue.

BM   What has the practice of yoga given you?

YM   Let's see…on the most crude level, on the most unspiritual level, it's one of the very few exercises I know – swimming is a little bit like it – where body and mind are linked.

At a more spiritual level, it helps to bring a sense of integrity, it helps unite you to something greater than yourself. Normally exercise, physical activity, tends to be somewhat egocentric: "my heart, my muscles, my strength, my appearance." There is something that I find wonderfully ego-destructive, in a positive sense, ego-loosening about yoga. Yoga isn't just some physical activity, it is part of a greater philosophy that has to be integrated into your life and that changes your life.

It is a wonderful way for people who are very reluctant to deal with spiritual matters. Sometimes for very good reasons, people who have been brought up in a very religious way rebel against that because of the errors of the Churches. Some people have a gut revulsion to anything spiritual. If you have suffered at the hands of religion, that has to be respected. Yoga, because in a sense the entry point is through the body, is a wonderful way to be spiritual but not in the way that balks some people in the West.

BM   You have traveled constantly since you were a child, yet you have said in the past that you can't live more than four years outside Canada. What is it about Canada that is so important to you?

YM   It's just where I am from. Aside from the fact that it is a wonderful country, it's a good country to live in, there's rule of law, the Canadian people are generous people, their social policies are generous. It's a very diverse place and it's a stunningly beautiful place. Aside from that, it is just where I am from. And you are where you are from. If I travel too long… I find if you travel more than six months, you start to drift a bit, you start to lose a sense of who you are and why you are.

Right now I love living in Saskatoon. I take daily pleasure in being in this country, in this city, with the people that I meet. The Prairies are stunning! There is a magical emptiness to it. You look upon it and you have to create and you want to fill that space. It's not a void, it's not a desert. It's most definitely not a desert. Maybe even deserts aren't what we think they are. There is something spiritual about these huge plains that is quite intoxicating – it really, really is.

BM   Give us a snapshot of your life as writer-in-residence at the Saskatoon Public Library.

YM   I work two days a week as a resource person. I am not here as a mentor and not here to teach creative writing. I am here to read people's stuff and just discuss it, to facilitate literary creativity in this community. I see people as young as fifteen and as old as late seventies. They come here to talk about their writing, words that they have invested themselves in, so I feel very privileged meeting with these people. Even if they lack artistry, it's nonetheless a moment where they are trying to express how they feel about this world, this universe, and I like that.

BM   Do you have any inklings or ambitions for where you would like to travel to next?

YM   Oh, God…have you got an hour for my list?! There are many ways of traveling, both physically, literally, in this world, but also in a mental way. As you get older you have to travel in different ways.

In my early twenties, I traveled in a completely carefree way, for no reason but just to see this big beautiful wide earth. Now because I am older I can't quite travel in that way. So now I travel with a purpose.

So, for example, three years ago I did the pilgrimage, the Road to St. James, the Santiago di Compostela. I walked across France and Spain. The idea of the pilgrimage appealed to me. Then after that I went to Portugal to do research for my next book, and when I was in Berlin I went to Poland to do the research for my next book. I usually have a purpose to my trip, usually research to do with a creative project.

I am not a travel writer, but traveling has definitely infused my creativity. To see different ways of being: whether it is different ways of speaking, different ways of eating, different ways of behaving with each other, of building cities, of transporting oneself. It just makes you aware of what a varied species we are. It's extraordinary. ॐ

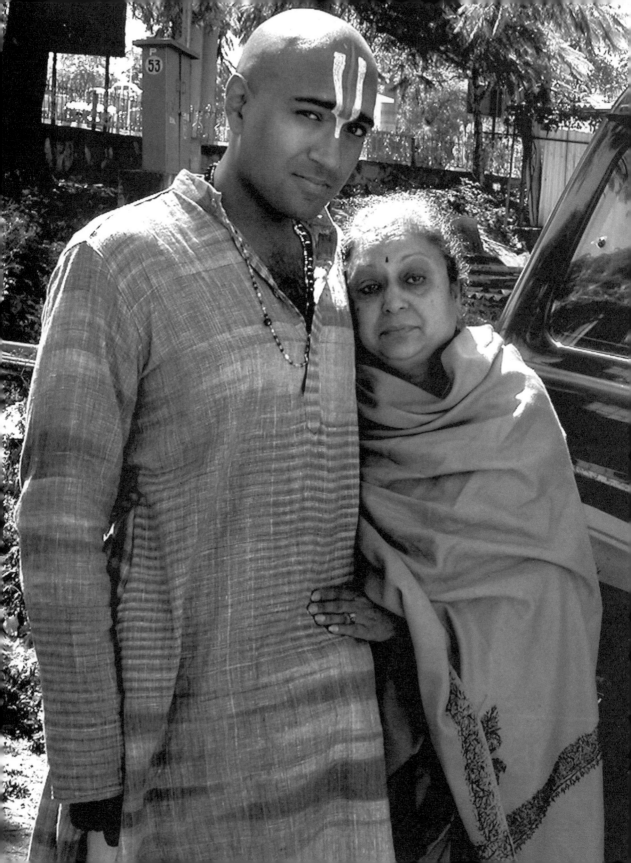

First published in Issue 22, Travel, Summer 2004

the cosmic current

can a pilgrimage really answer prayers?

[by Anand Ramayya]

my brother Raj, my filmmaking partner Tom and I traverse a staircase that winds its way up seven hills, nine miles and thousands of steps to the Tirupati Hill Shrine in Andhra Pradesh, southern India. The air thins and cools as we get higher and higher into the mountains. The stairs are lined with small tea stalls and soda vendors, spiced nuts at mile three. A *sadhu* is standing in the shade, steely-eyed, staring at us as we pass. His markings tell us his day began with prayer and the stillness of his eyes tells me I have a lot to learn.

We keep climbing.

The mid-morning heat is beating down, sweat pours and the stairs continue to unfold around every corner. With every step, I reflect on the past six weeks, the past year and indeed the past thirty years of my life. My mother was diagnosed with cancer last year and since then my family's world has changed. For the first time in twenty-five years we find ourselves in India together. As a family. And

film still courtesy of Anand Ramayya

I find myself somewhere I've never dreamed of, doing something I've never imagined ...

In the northern reaches of Saskatchewan in the boreal forest, the land of lakes, there exists a species indigenous to the deep south of India. Traditionally a non-smoking, non-drinking herbivore, upon migration the species has adopted North American feeding patterns and a potentially lethal obsession with filmmaking.

My name is Anand Ramayya, I am 100 percent South Indian–blooded, but I know absolutely nothing about what it means to be Indian. I was born and raised in Canada and grew up in the rugged but beautiful little town of La Ronge, Saskatchewan. Penumaka Dasarutha Ramayya and Jayalakshmi Presuna are my parents, descendants of a long line of orthodox Hindus with roots in southern India. My dad was a schoolteacher and my mom was a small-town girl when they married in 1965. Soon after, my brother Raj was born. The sixties was a time of opportunity for the educated immigrant, so my father and mother moved to Canada and re-invented themselves as Ray and Jaya Ramayya.

Ray has a Ph.D. in educational psychology and Jaya works at a daycare centre and sells Avon on the weekends. My father is obsessed with making films and my mother is equally determined to maintain some sense of normalcy in the household. She's stuck it out with him through three re-mortgages of the house and many other high-risk film financing stunts. While my dad has a knack for making things epic and complex, her strength is making things simple.

Like a lot of families these days, we've grown apart. My brother lives in Japan, I am constantly working and it seems none of us has had the time to get to know each other as adults. Life has a way of taking us so far from ourselves that everything gets blurry. This brush with mortality has focused us back in on the things that should matter. Things change when people get sick. I had originally planned to make a documentary about my father going to India to make his next film, but in the midst of it all my mother asked us to make a pilgrimage, as a family, to a place called Tirupati.

She's never asked us for anything. Ever.

With this one request, she has become a new person to me. A person with her own needs, with a past and a faith. None of which, I'm realizing, I know anything about.

India. Mystical, magical and overwhelming. The land of swamis, gurus and my family. At the airport, the customs officer shoots me a puzzled look and asks, "Are you Indian?" I don't quite know what to say. Two minutes later we are beeping and weaving our way through the freeway into the heart of the city.

Markets spill into the streets, traffic spills into the market and everything flows together. All of humanity seems to bubble over in the cauldron of Hyderabad. Beautiful minarets tower over us as we find our way into the heart of the Charminar Market. This was where my parents first lived after marriage. I feel myself transplanted in this new world where everything is chaotic and strange for me, yet for them it's home.

I am gaining a new kind of respect for my parents. I've taken them off the pedestal of parenthood and try to imagine myself in their position. I am six years older than my father and twelve years older than my mother when they had their first child. When they began with nothing and started to build their life, our life. It's a sobering and humbling thought. Had we stayed, I wonder who I would be in this India?

India is the seminal experience that is challenging the very foundation of my self-concept. Each moment is filled with meaning; each sight triggers a feeling or sensation that I didn't know existed in me. The indiscernible sound of locals slowly yields to my curious ears and becomes a language. A language I've only ever used unconsciously to listen in on household conversations is now connecting me to the 76 million people of this province.

I've romanticized this country in my dreams, but being here is a completely different story.

Each of us experiences our own India. For my father, India is a playground – a hustler's paradise. My sincere but self-indulgent moments of reflection are squished by his comic audacity. As I ponder my ultimate truths, he vanishes for hours only to reappear in the hotel lounge with a cellphone and some film cronies cooking up a deal. Andhra Pradesh does have the second-largest film industry in India.

But we remember that we are supposed to be here for my mother, to make a pilgrimage to pray for good health.

She steers us back toward family matters, and as we make our way I find new surprises around every corner, connections to a past I'd forgotten was mine.

When my brother finally arrives from Japan, we hit the road.

On my mother's list of stops is a visit to the home of my wise little uncle in Hyderabad who wakes up at four a.m. to listen to classical Indian music and perform his prayers to Jesus, Allah, Buddha, Sai Baba and Venkateswara. "They are all the same – there is only one God," he declares matter-of-factly as he inches his way past me to his morning pot of ginger tea. He is quite a contrast to my father, who wakes every morning to a cigarette, cup of coffee and copy of *American Cinematographer.* Uncle's home is peaceful and in his bedroom there is a picture of Venkateswara Swami, the presiding deity of Tirupati. I ask him why people go to Tirupati.

"People have desires, so by doing a pilgrimage they can have their wishes answered."

"And why do people shave their heads and give their hair in Tirupati?" I ask.

"It is only a belief and we offer it to the Lord," says Uncle.

This extremely slight and charming eighty-five-year-old creaks from room to room conserving energy for more entertaining endeavours, such as his daily prayers, complaining about the news and today, giving his youngest brother, my father, a hard time. My father wants a better answer.

"Why? Why do they offer?" my father demands.

"What do you mean? What is the belief? What am I supposed to tell you? If you believe, then there is the belief, that's it. Are you following me?"

I am following him, slowly but surely.

The next morning we are on our way to my mother's childhood home of Eluru. Pavement drops to dirt, cows and goats decide to share the road with us. We go deeper and deeper into Andhra Pradesh. The farther we go, the more I realize how little I know about my mother.

We enter her hometown and it is like a snapshot from the past. I can see her as a little girl living in this neighbourhood and playing on these streets. Streets that haven't changed much since her days.

We walk along a narrow dusty street lined with clay and brick pastel-coloured homes. It has been twelve years since she last visited and twenty-five years since her family has seen her two sons. Without hesitation, we are welcomed into her old home and another piece of her past.

"My mother passed away when I was four, around thirteen my father passed away," she tells me. "I lived here first eighteen years of my life. My aunt brought me up and gave me a good education and good advice and put me through schools and dancing schools. But still I felt, I wish I have my mom and dad.

"When I go through my tough times, bad times, good times, I always think about God and my mom and dad. That is the soothing thing for my stress points. When I think about my health problems or financial problems, everything goes when you look at God, pictures and your grandparents and everything. I feel soothing things for me all around."

It is hard for her to talk about these things. I can see my mother was really happy here, but the walls are filled with memories and emotion.

Seeing her here, I feel she is definitely from this place and in some ways maybe she's never left. The ease of laughter, her comfort with friends, the unspoken understandings between them – she glides through India. She's one of these women, enforcers of the moral code that binds the Indian family system. Their patience, strength and beliefs seem to hold their families together.

I decide to consult a swami before heading out on the last leg to Tirupati. I have a lot of unanswered questions. I wait in his receiving hall, the walls lined with photos, deities and garlands. The clock ticks, time stands still and my mind races. Why am I here? What is it that I'm looking for? Who could possibly answer any of these questions? At this moment I can't imagine myself being any further away from anywhere I ever thought I would be.

I am told to begin with my questions.

I take a deep breath, try to suspend my cynicism and begin.

"Swami-ji. Who am I?"

"Who am I, who am I? This is good question. Suppose anybody comes and asks you, who are you? You should not say I am an Indian, I am an American, I am Canadian, I am a Hindu, I am a Christian. First of all bravely you must say, I am a human being. If all the people on the Earth can bravely say that they are human beings, having perfect humanity, then the whole Earth becomes peaceful."

"What is God and how do you define God?" I ask.

"According to me, there is only one God, who is omnipresent and omnipotent," says the swami. "There is only one religion and that is the religion of love. Who is God, where is God and what is the form of God? God is the cosmic current which is pervading through every atom of the universe. It is everywhere, in everybody, in every atom, it is just like current flowing."

It takes me awhile to appreciate his words, but ultimately I realize that I have to let go of my expectations and just allow myself to be. My family in India seems to share similar values of tolerance, peace and a connection to an omnipresent God whose name, shape and size is irrelevant. Jesus, Allah, Buddha, Venkateswara. They are all the same.

I am starting to realize that understanding the spirituality of India is the key to understanding my mother, and maybe even a bit of myself.

The Muslims have Mecca, the Christians have Jerusalem, but for Hindus, Tirupati is the holiest of holy places, the transcendental plane on Earth where my ancestors have gone for generations to have their prayers granted. The ancient sages of India believed the rigorous walk up these seven hills would fulfill the vows of the pilgrim. They believed that the essence of God is held inside this temple. God, the Soul and the Universe together form one reality. An all-pervading cosmic current.

We have traveled across the world to make this pilgrimage and walk these steps up to the ancient and sacred temple of Sri Venkateswara on the seventh peak of Tirupati Hill. The town and the hills are bursting with the energy of the 50,000 pilgrims that come here daily.

It was my mother's will that brought us here, but ironically her body isn't strong enough to walk the steps. My father stays behind with her and only the young in our group start on the trek.

We are an unlikely crew from the other side of the planet. Me, my brother freshly unplugged from the Tokyo club scene, and Tom, who is sporting a mini-DV camera and sunscreen. We aren't exactly blending in with the other pilgrims, but each of us has our own appointment in these sacred hills. For some reason, fate has brought us here, thousands of miles from home.

We keep walking, mile after mile, step after step. The equipment seems to get heavier as the air thins. Our machismo fades as my three young cousins glide by us and giggle. We stop for spiced pineapple and catch our breath. After mile four everything becomes about breathing. All I can hear is my breath and I can see clearly that the place I am in is magic.

For a moment on these hills, I allow myself to believe in something bigger than myself. That somehow by performing this ritual I can defy all logic and compel this inexplicable universal power to transform my world, answer my prayers. That somehow at the end of this path there is a chance for liberation and a merger, perhaps, with God and the universe.

The ancient sages believed shaving one's head is an act of complete surrender of your ego at the feet of the Lord. It is also my final step in a pilgrimage that has taken me from my hometown of La Ronge to this Transcendental Plane on Earth. The blade scrapes my scalp, stroking away the weight of my thoughts. We are all tired, it has been a long road, but this moment is so simple, so absolute.

And regardless of whether I believe in my mother's God or not, I respect her faith. She has been coming here since she was a child. And I do believe that the act of this pilgrimage is real for her, that God exists in this temple and that the act of the pilgrimage itself has fulfilled all of her wishes.

For now, that's all I need. ॐ

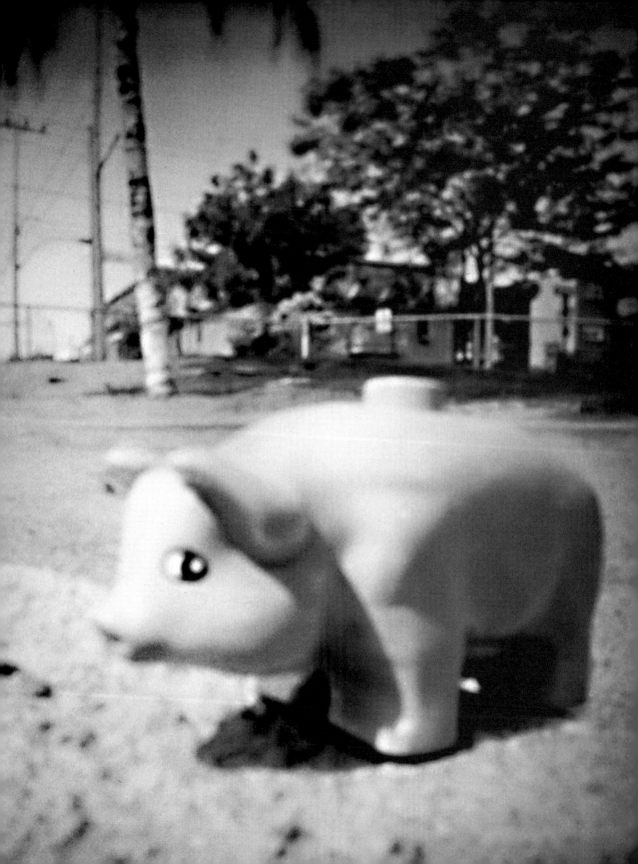

First published in Issue 19, Myth & Storytelling, Fall 2003

the origami of found objects

"to restore silence is the role of objects" – Samuel Beckett

[by Catherine Kidd]

there was this plastic pig. It was found in a Lost and Found box, on the basement floor of the Jewish Y, near the kindergarten rooms. The pig was about the size of an Aspirin bottle, and had been there for weeks. Every Sunday afternoon, when I went to yoga class in the kindergarten, I saw it lying at the bottom of the box among odd mitts.

I eventually assumed the pig was lost, so I found it. I stuck the pig in the front pocket of my pack, and from then on it went with me everywhere. Sometimes I took out the pig and looked at it, rolled it in my palm or set it on a table. I wasn't sure what it represented yet, but I seemed to care about the pig. It wore an expression of keen but humble curiosity, glancing sidelong.

When my friend and I went for spinach pizza at Terrasse Lafayette, the pig sat on the table. At one point, when I returned from the washroom, my friend had constructed a tent for the pig, out of a napkin. The pig's head was peeking out of it; the tent was not very big. When we left the restaurant, I tucked the napkin tent

photo by C. Caruso

into my bag, with the pig.

You're going to keep the pig-tent? It's just a scrap of folded paper.

My friend was laughing because he was not surprised. I do this. I save things. It is partly due to an old and hereditary conviction that I will not be able to remember events properly unless I have some tangible evidence that they might have occurred. A plastic pig or a paper tent can act as a mnemonic device, a talisman to summon clairvoyant images of some past time and place. They can recreate a sense-experience of memory, carrying smell, carrying texture, perhaps conducting energy.

Or maybe it's simply that I persist in believing the napkin will feel depressed if I abandon it, a conviction some might view as a bit of a problem. But surely a crumpled napkin, like the rest of creation, is as sentient and sensitive as its observer. I am a storyteller, and for a storyteller, this belief or sensibility is somewhat essential. Things do not have to be factual to be true.

My father was similarly afflicted. He collected objects he found on the street, everything from swizzle sticks to odd tires. Each object seemed to have a sort of ritual significance to him, corresponding to its shape or location, or some symbolic meaning. I remember a wooden box he kept on his dresser, where there was a pipe-cleaner bumble bee inside a plastic Aspirin container, which he called his *Let it Bee*. There was also an orange origami crane, a tiny goat knitted out of string, and a cast-iron rugby player who kicked at a ball when you pressed a lever on his crown cakra.

If, one day, a person were to unfold the origami crane, she might be able to figure out how it was made. After some trial and error, she might be able to recreate it newly.

This is how memory works. Mine anyway, and apparently my father's. It attaches itself to objects and unfolds them, to take in the rest of the room, the gradual details of past time and place. In this way, all objects can be origami cranes. You can unfold them, and in their creases trace the path of their coming to be. Through the interaction between hands and paper, inanimate objects become animate. They become legible; they tell a story.

Looking at this pig now, I think what it represents to me is patience. Maybe it's the expression on its face, its gentle curiosity, or the fact that the pig sat in this mess of lost objects for weeks, while I gradually learned how to stretch and breathe, next door in the kindergarten room. This learning was gradual, and cumulative, like evolution. It required patience, the ability to be engaged in a process of situating oneself. Eventually, I found this pig, although I'd known it was there all along.

It's significant, too, that my friend felt urged to build a makeshift napkin house for the pig, as though a sense of home were the only missing ingredient from the story I was implicitly writing. My friend understands me fairly well. There is something about the writing and telling of stories that is closely connected to notions of exile and belonging, of losing oneself and finding oneself.

> My storehouse having
> Burnt down,
> Nothing obscures
> My view
> Of the bright moon.
> – Zen poem

Like finding something, losing something has transformative power. Stories are often generated from a sense of loss, middling through the process of mourning, cresting with the act of chronicling, taking stock, bearing witness, holding accountable. And, more often than not, ending in a sense of renewal and recovery. Evolution occurs here, spontaneously. Something new is found, the missing thing becoming tangible in the story itself.

It may be impossible to extract any single most influential event in one's artistic life, when every event seems, in retrospect, so part of a process. But if asked, I'd probably say that my destined choice to be a storyteller has much to do with my father. I'd mention the letters he wrote to me during the last months of his life, and the sad fact that he died before we could be properly reconciled. And that he very much wished to open up correspondence between us during the last two years of his life.

I was in India at the time. Sometimes I'd find a letter at the Benares Poste Restante, and learn that he lived in a trailer with a three-legged hamster named Dusty, or that he'd been collecting bottles and cans from the beach in Gibsons, BC, in a shopping cart. Or that they'd been siphoning fluid from his abdomen to control his cancer. Or sometimes the letters were letters from God, as transcribed by my father.

My father, his own description, spoke in tongues. This meant that he frequently went into a semblance of trance, and uttered words that appeared nonsensical. Or unfamiliar, at least. When I was a teenager, this was extremely embarrassing to me. Despite my interest in religious studies, part of me couldn't completely believe in it. I wished I could, but it was the early eighties and I wore my hair short and cynical. My father seemed quaint, eccentric, exasperating.

It has only been in more recent years that I realize we have far more in common than I was ever willing to admit while he was alive. For a long time, this was a source of great sadness. But today, when I think of how he described this state of being, where he perceived himself primarily as a vessel for some story to come forth – some utterance that he was the channel for, but not the owner of – it makes perfect sense to me. It is very similar to the experience of telling a story. There is a sort of surrender involved, a relinquishment of ownership.

Instead of assuming control, when I'm performing, I have found rather the opposite to occur: a giving over of control to the story itself. It has always felt more true to say that the stories perform me than vice versa. This is not a supernatural thing, but simply the result of an identification with the action rather than the actor. The self becomes more a vessel or conduit than a discrete entity when it is acting in accordance with its own life purpose, and speaking from that place. *Is this similar to speaking in tongues?*

But there's this, too. It might be loopy to think that stories are floating around in the atmosphere, and that the artist is some sort of magnetic earthly mouthpiece for them. Yet I've noticed that many artists describe creative process as a kind of surrender, a willingness to be led by a certain energy or volition, which is the unfolding of work itself. The artist journeys through the looking glass, and enters that magical state called *creative process*. Conversations with others become full of answers to the exact questions one has been asking the universe, and objects found on the sidewalk carry the enhanced resonance of objects in dreams. The human becomes willing to engage in an ongoing story, and the artist becomes pregnant in some way.

The other day I bought a Kinder egg, one of those chocolate eggs with a prize inside a plastic orange capsule, and usually some assembly required. Inside my egg, and after assembly, I found a blue and yellow caterpillar taking a bath inside a pink open lotus flower, one of her several limbs holding a scrub brush. The caterpillar reminds me of Lakshmi, mother of creative energy, bringing gifts of health and prosperity. If the pig was saddled with a reputation for being a bit untidy, here was a creature who was cleaning herself up, in process of transformation into something with wings.

But do I believe that some Divine power or unearthly relative caused me to choose the particular egg with the caterpillar inside, in the knowledge that this object would carry some significance for me? I would have to say no, because too often similar excuses of Divine instruction are used to justify misguided choices.

Do I think the caterpillar is a sign of some sort? Yes, I choose to. It may well be that the primary function of choice is the manner in which experiences are read. Like the caterpillar who met Alice with the question, "So you think you're changed, do you?" my caterpillar arrived at the threshold of a certain process of change, and seems to wear an expression of genuine astonishment at the fact.

A typo of not long ago produced the phrase *praying attention*. The *r* was accidental and unconscious, but a private evolution seemed to occur instantaneously. I could continue to choose remorse and regret for the fact that I missed the opportunity to have a relationship with my father during the last years of his life. This would inspire stories of remorse and regret, and I might get stuck there, believing what I read and have written. And so, eventually, I came to choose otherwise. There is a gift contained in patience, and even in grief. It is choice that eventually unwraps the gift, and is grateful, and through gratitude evolves. ॐ

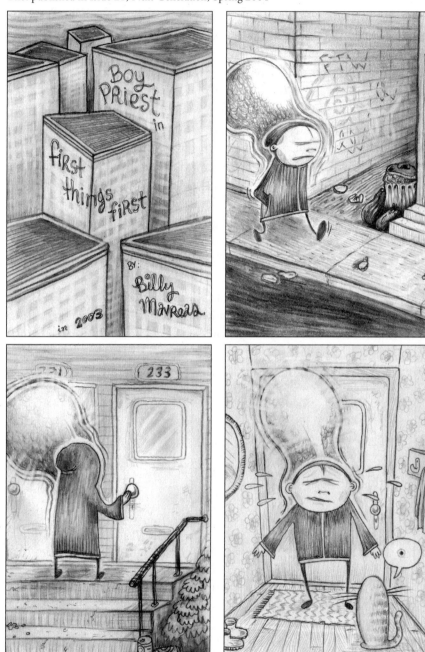

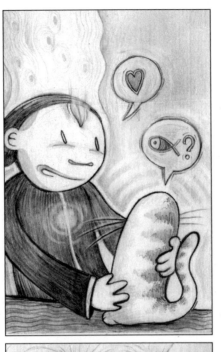
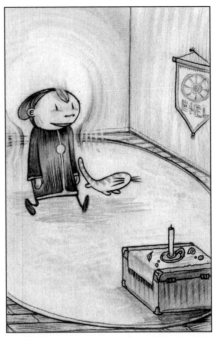
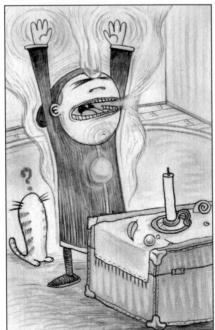
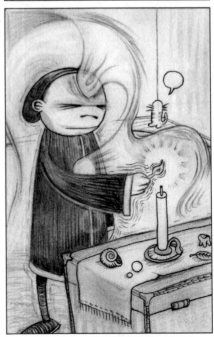

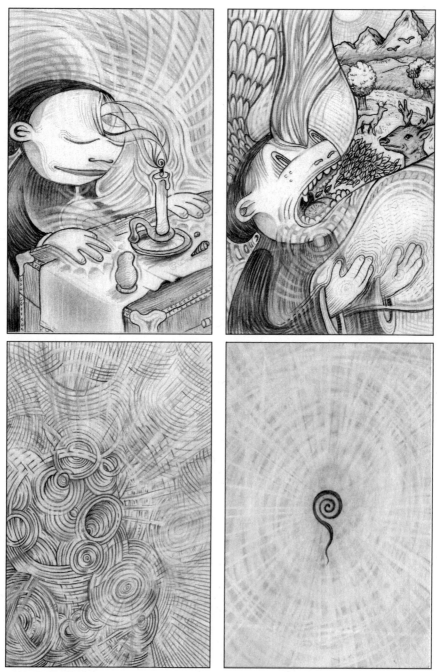

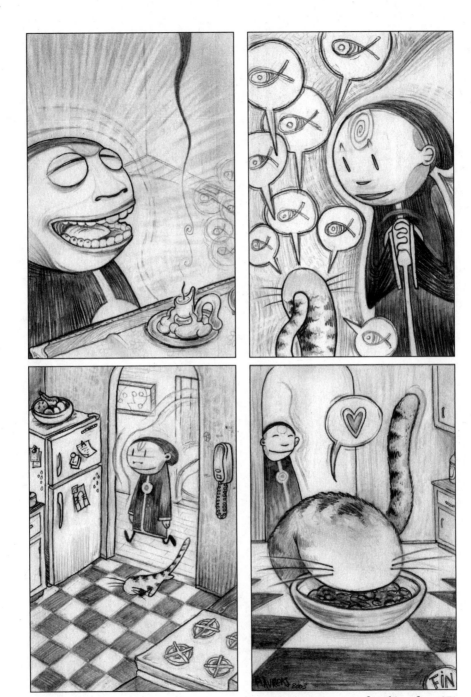

I look in the mirror and wonder, "Who am I? What is my self, without my social props and book collection?" I am like Descartes, who closed his eyes, removed all his possessions, and asked, "Do I exist?"

First published in Issue 22, Travel, Summer 2004

my visit to california
fragments of travel

[by Sparrow]

because I live in a mountain town, I ride a bus into New York City to board an airplane to California. On the bus from Phoenicia to Manhattan, I wrote the following: I enjoy watching a man read – it is often as engaging as reading oneself. *Nathaniel's Story* by Anne Whitehead is what the man in front of me holds in his hand.[1]

With his other hand (his right), he caresses his moustache. Then at times he rests this hand on his lip.

He reads slowly, drawn into the imaginary story.

The way he touches his facial hair is almost seductive. My wife touches my beard like that on certain nights.

Reading is self-romance. You believe two people in your chapter kiss, but really you are falling in love with yourself.

I learned all this from watching a man with a moustache read.

There is no longer food service on airplanes! Even American Airlines! Instead, one collects a tiny paper bag containing a sandwich and a bag of miniature carrots, as one enters the plane. The stewardesses content themselves with endlessly serving drinks.

Lake Michigan, from above, is as limitless as the Indian Ocean. Dipping down to enter Chicago, I suddenly see synchronized waves on its surface – appearing miniature, like 400 choreographed grasshopper legs dancing.

At the Chicago airport: people are fatter. In the middle of America bodies are larger than at the edges.

From Chicago to San Jose, I have a seat with no window. This is a lengthy flight, too – four hours and six minutes! And all I brought to read was a strange memoir by George Sand, *Winter in Majorca*. I begin to panic about the long span of time. I tell the woman next to me, "I am about to meditate. If you need to use the bathroom, just tap me on the shoulder."

I close my eyes. An announcement comes over the intercom: "We will soon begin our feature presentation for this flight, *Johnny English*."

Thank God! They'll show a movie!

I open my eyes and buy a headset for two dollars.

I forgot – here in America the longest one goes without entertainment is twenty minutes.

My hotel in San Jose is so luxurious the bathroom has a television! Its five-inch screen faces the shower. Curious, I turn it on. The picture is black and white, and rolls. Nonetheless, it does depict a lovable monster movie.

Also in the bathroom is a large convex mirror, which magnifies my face enormously, so that I may apply makeup. (I discover this abruptly as I rise from the toilet.)

I stow my backpack in the closet. Then I check the drawer of my nightstand for the Bible – but I don't open it. For years I opened the Bible at random as an oracle each time I found it, until once, on a visit to Albany (New York), I turned to the death of Solomon, and became convinced I was going to be hit by a car.

I lie on my firm bed and close my eyes. *I am on the wrong side of the continent*, I feel. This is a disjointed sensation, as if I had just had a knee operation and the doctor removed my kidney by mistake.

Hanging in my closet is a white belted bathrobe (on a hanger) with a hotel insignia. On an impulse I wear it, hoping to resemble Sherlock Holmes. Instead, in the mirror I see an inept middle-aged karate instructor.

I walk out into the San Jose air. Everything is warm, and I become somehow liquid. I feel the street drinking me.

I see the license plate: ENJLIF

(That must mean "Enjoy Life.")

Perhaps because I am on vacation, everyone seems to be on vacation; no one carries a purse or bag. All the citizens walk freely, and smile.

Early in *Winter in Majorca*, George Sand considers the meaning of travel:

The fact is that nowhere, these days, is anyone genuinely happy, and that of the countless faces assumed by the Ideal – or, if you dislike the word, the concept of something better – travel is one of the most engaging and most deceitful. All is rotten in public affairs: those who deny this truth feel it even more deeply and bitterly than those who assert it. Nevertheless, divine Hope still pursues her way, assuaging our tormented hearts with the constant whisper, "There is something better – namely, your ideal!"

Our social order does not even command the sympathies of its defenders; each of us in dissatisfaction chooses whatever escape suits him best. One throws himself into art, another into science, the majority stupefy themselves with whatever comes nearest to hand. All of us who have time and money to spare, travel – that is to say, we flee; since surely it is not so much a question of traveling as of getting away?

I am surprised how much I *do* escape myself, when I travel. So much of my "self" is my house, with its sofa, dining table, garbage can, foods. My friends and companions constitute much of my "self." My work also creates "me." I would say that on my trip to California 80 percent of "me" stayed behind and 20 percent left.

For one thing, I become younger when I travel. The alert, curious and ignorant mind I have is exactly like my mind at eighteen. Which means that on my travels the year is 1972. This is especially true of places like San Jose, where some of 1972 does linger.

The word "vacation" means "the act of vacating" – in other words, creating a void. There is a void at my house, where my wife and daughter continue without me, and also a void inside me. I travel as a moving void.

There is so much to learn when you travel – and much of this is spatial learning. When I reached my hotel room, for example, I couldn't find the pitcher and glasses they promised me. I searched throughout my two rooms, but couldn't discover it. Finally, I called the desk. A friendly woman answered. "They're inside the television chest," she explained.

Of course! I do not watch television, so I don't open that chamber!

Next, I walked the hall until I found the filtered water dispenser. (The man at the desk had candidly admitted the unfiltered water was horrible.) All this spatial searching is like the learning one does at age three and four. (In which case, the year is 1957.)

When traveling, each moment devours the previous one. As I watched *Johnny English,* the comic intelligence of Rowan Atkinson captivated me. Immediately after, I became consumed with curiosity about the woman on my left who was reading *O* magazine [produced by Oprah]. Had she bought the magazine, or found it somehow on the plane? And if she *had* bought the magazine, why? Was she a follower of Oprah, or did she buy it at random? (Come to think of it, the flight originated in Chicago – Oprah's city – so perhaps her magazine was prominently displayed.) Was this woman a *liberal* (like Oprah)?

In my anonymous room, wearing my bland traveling clothes, I look in the mirror and wonder, "Who am I? What is my self, without my social props and book collection?" I am like Descartes, who closed his eyes, removed all his possessions, and asked, "Do I exist?"[2]

I lie down on my bed and turn on the clock radio. I find the station KSTU; a young woman is playing "Get out of My Car" by a local group called Imaginary Girlfriend. I like this song – a neo-garage rushing three-chord plea. So, this is a clue to my personality. I am someone who enjoys Imaginary Girlfriend.

There is value to this knowledge.

At any moment a new friend may appear – at least a temporary friend – in travel. Someone may stop to ask directions who stays at your hotel. In a tavern, the man next to you may begin talking about his wife.

I walk among my many possible friends.

My favourite part of hotel travel is the free soap I receive. At the Isla Vista, the bar was rather large (for free soap) and oval. I carry a plastic bag to deposit the soap in, so it will not wet my backpack. Thus protected, I carry the soap 2994 miles, back to Phoenicia. There my family will wash with it, until it finally dissolves.

A voyage is always a beginning – even a trip to a cemetery. As you climb the steps of the bus, you feel you are in a movie. You can almost hear the jaunty clarinets and strings behind you. The movie is beginning, and you are the hero! ॐ

---

[1] I fish my eyeglasses out of my bag to see the title. This is the only purpose my glasses serve.
[2] His answer was, "*Je pense, donc je suis*" – "I think, thus I am."

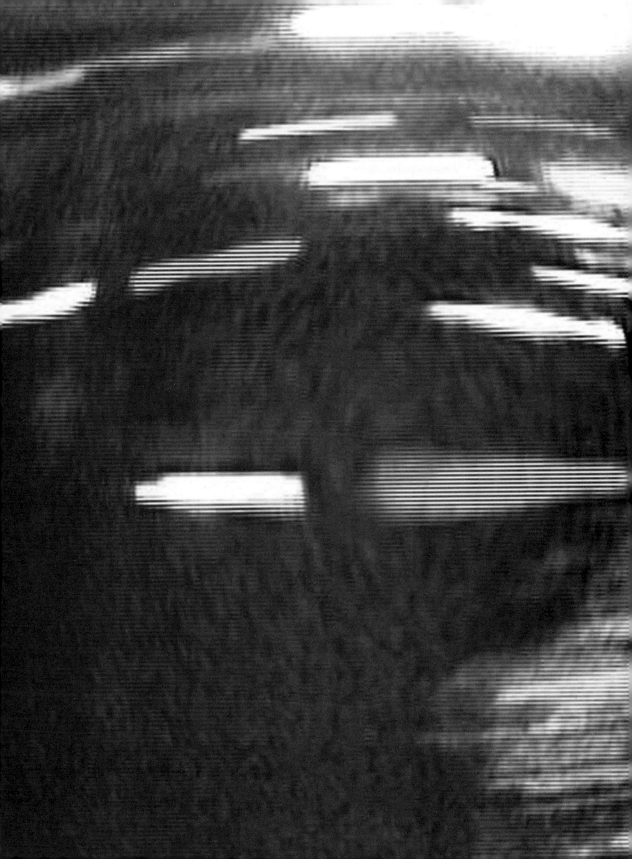

First published in Issue 22, Travel, Summer 2004

this prayer wheel we spin
on tour with the automated prayer machine

[by Annabelle Chvostek]

it is early February and a light snow covers the Eastern European countryside. We pass through low mountains and forests, past the tiled roofs of old villages. Castles sit majestically atop high rocky perches. New developments tear through the mountains, grey apartment buildings teetering on the brink of the factories they exist to serve. The hard edges of Communist functionality seem strangely at odds with the medieval towns that circle outward from their highest points of church and state.

Departing from Vienna, I am moving through the Czech landscape toward Prague. Anna Friz sits across from me as the train passes through cities, towns and countryside. We head toward our last stops on a month-long European tour to present our collaboration, a new media musical performance called *The Automated Prayer Machine*.

Fate has me traveling toward Slovakia, the landscape of my father's heritage, as he, across the ocean, prepares to embark upon a six-hour open-heart surgery,

video still courtesy of Annabelle Chvostek

scheduled in a few days' time. I got word of his imminent procedure in Vienna at the Kunstradio studio, immediately after our live broadcast on Austrian national radio. The news hit like a ton of bricks. Thankfully, I have a focus for the unfurling emotions. The music of the *Prayer Machine* is constantly purring through my body – the building layers of violin harmonies, swooping satellite sounds, the enveloping drone of accordion. Snippets of its wise words spill into my mind, and I know that I will be performing with a heightened passion.

Anna and I created *The Automated Prayer Machine* as an antidote to the bombardment of disturbing news – to broadcast hope, inspiration, potential. With our mutual love of electronic soundscape and traditional musical instruments, we set forth to perform a prayer wheel. We asked our friends and communities to send prayers by email or to record messages on our answering machines. Their replies became the fabric in a concert of live radio transmissions that, when performed, takes us on a challenging voyage toward a destination of rippling sound and lighted words.

When we first put out the call for prayers, we had no idea how it would be received. I pressed "send" to an email list of hundreds, with a Ganesh mantra on the brain, but part of me was cynical, if curious and hopeful. Who prays these days? And how do they do it? The answering machine messages started pouring in almost immediately. As we digitized them, I could feel my heart centre moving. One of those rare glimpses of opening that almost tickles with a tear-jerking bliss.

The nervous jitters, the dim lights, the hush of the room. The Automated Prayer Machine *performance begins with blips of short-wave radio noise bouncing through the space on portable radios that have been placed throughout the audience. Anna and I sit behind a table full of wires, samplers, effects pedals and mixers. The noise builds. This is our Radio Tower of Babel, the darkest moment in the piece, when we stir up the silt of the last few years of terror-heavy media reports and face the scourge of right-wing talk radio. We are taking a furious ride through a sonic climate of sensationalism, airing the stuff that makes us fearful and apathetic. Anna captures live radio and feeds it into a pulsating mass. I throw in snapshot samples of wild street drumming.*

"I'm talkin' about war," says the twangy fundamentalist preacher.

For this we pick up our instruments and pound out a tchardas, *Anna on*

her accordion, and I with my violin, starting in time to a rhythm of words, a slow
minor oompah, old country in the blood. Gradually we speed into a dancing frenzy.
No longer numbed by the media, we stop … and drop into a heartbeat of looping
accordion.

We step off the subway and into downtown Prague, met by the wide and bustling grandeur of Wenceslas square. Angels on chariots with gilded wings scan the scene from high atop the national museum. Capitalism tacks itself adolescently onto the facades of the grand old stately buildings. I must have my brow furrowed, life-and-death thoughts jumbling through the brain.

"I pray for an end to worrying," said one of our call-in prayers.

My strong dad. Just before we left, he'd been vigorously fixing my exploding water pipes after a vicious Montréal cold snap. Nobody knew how serious it was, that a valve in his heart was malfunctioning, that his lungs were slowly filling up with fluid.

"It seems like such a strange fulfillment that we should be heading to Slovakia right now, like the whole trip has been pointing us east to this moment. Who knows, it might be the most profound thing you can do for your dad," says Anna.

"If you need to go back, though, I'll help in any way I can."

I can't think. I'm busy trying not to cry in public. We go eat dumplings in spinach sauce with sauerkraut and beer. It's good.

We wander through the old town and venture along the famous Charles Bridge, which lines the passage across the wide Danube river with vivid and gory illusionist baroque tableaux. Cast in bronze and carved out of blackening stone – there are crosses carried, crosses hung upon, despairing Marys and saint upon Catholic saint.

We step off the bridge and through its majestic gateway tower, toward the maze of medieval streets now bursting with tourist shops, restaurants and puppet theatres. I need to make a phone call. On the Gothic streets of old Prague, overlooked by buildings dripping with statuary – angels ready to take flight from the rooftops, monks reading, cherubs playing, Hercules holding up the architecture – I talk to my pre-op dad in his hospital bed.

I ask him if I should come home early. I'm faced with the fact that he might not survive the surgery. But he is positive, wanting me to finish my tour and perform in Slovakia. And, in a way, it makes perfect sense. Perhaps this prayer wheel we spin has found its truest intention within this urgent moment. I have an opportunity to focus healing and collaborate with the highest good. I want my brilliant father to continue living. And if he cannot, I want him to fly with ease, with joy.

Even budget apartments in Prague have sculpted Grecian faces above the tall wooden doorways. It is our last night here and we spend it jamming with our hosts, Steven and Hanna. I'm ridiculously overjoyed as Hanna brings life to old Slovak songs that I pull out of my memory banks. Her grandmother was a singer and the songs have been passed along. Hanna says the best music comes from Slovakia and Moravia, all the saddest, most beautiful melodies. She teaches us lilting medieval modes, tales of sisters searching for brothers gone to war, of lovers and flower gardens.

Part two of The Automated Prayer Machine *is* The Requiem. *We are bathed in the blue-green light of video projection. A huge school of fish swims in barely perceptible slow motion across the screen. We build loops with our instruments until a pleading orchestral intensity emerges and swells. Then the video fades into an image of the low wall around the main stupa at Bodh Gaya. It is covered in a stream of hundreds of brightly burning candles. The mood breaks and shifts into gentle shimmering hope.*

The train rushes silent through the countryside. Inside, the cars are full yet hushed. Outside is the stillness of winter. We are on our way to Slovakia. In half an hour, my father's surgery will start. I stare out the window and begin to pray in earnest. Hours pass as I watch the landscape shift and unfold. I am focused, receiving, transmitting.

Woods, low mountains and jutting rocks fall away into the flatlands of my grandfather's Moravia – field upon field interrupted only by small groupings of trees and tiny houses. This is the land in between. Something happens here. Hares leap across the landscape, flying on their strong hind legs. Groupings of deer bound through the fields, white tails upturned. Something surreal and magical is going on. The voice inside is exclaiming, "Life!"

I entered this journey with Anna to find out what it meant to pray in this crazy modern world, hoping for a channel to emerge. The prayers we have gathered and broadcast, the people we have connected with, have brought me to this moment. The wheel is spinning and I am coming home.

We arrive in Bratislava, the ancient capital of Slovakia, and have a few hours before my mother calls with the word. After lugging our gear to the hotel, we wander outside into a fresh light snowfall, lured by the pretty stuccoed buildings, the curving streets and the sound of music. We're drawn to the central square where a band is playing a robust Balkan *ska*. People are dancing, eating and drinking. We catch the last chord and go looking for a good meal and a shot of Slivovic, a strong plum brandy, the smell of which still evokes my grandmother's china cabinet.

As we curve back through the cobblestones, the city is alive. My inner voice says "STABLE" and I want to believe it, but I continue to silently freak out until I hear my mother's voice on the phone. She calls me as soon as I get in. "His heart rate is stable, his blood is stable, his oxygen level is stable, everything is stable. They couldn't repair the valve so they replaced it with a pig valve. You're dad's not kosher anymore," she jokes. She has been through a day of hell. She is relieved and exhausted. Dad is hooked up to a million machines. But hallelujah, he is stable.

It's Saturday and the town square is hopping once again. A horn quintet plays ethereally and later stilt-walkers with huge folk-art masks meander throughout pockets of people. We laugh as a skeletal grim reaper approaches us. What else can you do?

That night the show goes well, the venue, A-4, is gorgeous, our hosts are lovely, the poster is cool. We dedicate our performance to my pa, back home, unconscious and wired up, but emerging.

Part three is our namesake, The Automated Prayer Machine, *woven out of the response to our call for prayers. Armed with Anna's tiny twelve-watt transmitter, an armada of radios and scores of heartfelt wishes, we spin the prayers out into space in concentric waves of radio. On the video screen the gentle light of a wintry city night turns and turns. Our instruments whirr, making loops of soft mechanical harmonics.*

"I pray for some good ideas... to make the world a better place..."

"...Where there is despair, hope."

"May sunlight shine upon you and warm your heart, until it glows like a great peat fire, so that strangers may come and warm themselves by it."

"May every creature abound in well-being and peace...weak or strong, the long and the small, the short and the medium-sized, the mean and the great."

"I pray that I realize how lucky I really am."

There are blessings, beatitudes and mantras. There is a hilarious prayer to the "Goddess, you anarchist slut," a prayer to Brigitte of the Mountain, an Aramaic Lord's prayer and a prayer to the morning. There are personal prayers for courage and accountability, for the wild things, for refugees, for an end to greed, for the women of Vancouver's Lower East Side. There are abundant prayers for peace. By the middle of our trip, we have prayers in Flemish, Finnish, German, Italian, Hindi, Croatian, Spanish and Pharisee.

A professor once taught me that there are as many forms of Hinduism as there are Hindus. I would venture to say that there are as many forms of prayer as there are people praying. Prayer found me when I needed it. It was like stepping into a void, swimming within the light and flow of some shifting parallel world. I can't pin it down, but somehow entering its infinite potential is possible. Switch it on and let the transmission fly.

It's my sixth day back in Canada. As I write this, Dad is plucking on his mandolin, laughing with the family. One whole lot of love is going on. "Life! Life is good," he said earlier today in his first hour home from the hospital.

More than ever, I know that death will come for all of us. But for now, oh Cosmic Birther of all radiance and vibration, we've got some good living to do. ॐ

about the contributors

Marcus Boon teaches contemporary literature at York University in Toronto. He is the author of *The Road of Excess: A History of Writers on Drugs* (Harvard UP 2003). His writings can be found at www.hungryghost.net. He is currently researching a history of twentieth-century writers involved with Asian spiritual practices, entitled *Sadhana*.

Brent Burbridge is a researcher and writer living in Toronto.

Annabelle Chvostek is a musician, composer, videographer and singer/songwriter living in Montréal. She writes, tours and records extensively, and is a member of roots songwriter collective The Wailin' Jennys. For information on her projects and performances, see www.annabelle.org.

Jeffry Farell investigates the nature of Presence via the performing arts, teaching and yoga. Practising since the 1970s, he owns Aha Yoga and Health Center in Dallas, Texas, where he teaches daily. His investigations into Presence have carried him through realms of elegant slapstick, tragic choruses, festive rebellions and mysterious joys. He's married with children ages one, four, and sixteen, who keep his attention present. Kumar Pallana remains his primary yoga teacher.

Juniper Glass is a Montréal writer, yoga student and teacher, and community animator. In 2003–2004, she was *ascent* magazine's managing editor. Originally from British Columbia, she studied international development at the University of Guelph and yoga in Bombay and Kootenay Bay. Some of her favourite things these days are family life, Rilke's *Book of Hours,* dancing, and understanding jokes in French. Reach her at juniperglass@hotmail.com.

Soren Gordhamer is a thirty-seven-year-old husband, father, writer and meditation teacher. He is founder of the Lineage Project, an innovative nonprofit organization that teaches meditation and yoga to incarcerated and at-risk teens in New York City. A winner of the Mayor's Voluntary Action Award from former NYC mayor Rudolph Giuliani, the Lineage Project has worked with youth in juvenile halls, prisons and community centres. Soren is also the author of the meditation book for teens *Just Say OM!* (Adams Media, 2001). A graduate of Spirit Rock Meditation Center's "Community Dharma Leaders Program," Soren has taught classes for teens in numerous environments, including drug rehabilitation programs, juvenile halls, private high schools and community classes.

Sikeena Karmali was born in Nairobi, Kenya to Gujarati Indian parents. She was educated in Canada, the US, Italy and Egypt. Since 1994 she has worked in international development and human rights, and was recently the director of a human rights agency in Tashkent, Uzbekistan. She lives in Vancouver and is working on her second novel about journeys of the Silk Road. She is also a contributing editor at *ascent* magazine.

Catherine Kidd is the author/performer of *Sea Peach,* a CD/book collection of stories as well as a critically acclaimed stage show. Described as "an adult blend of Dr. Seuss and Aesop's Fables," *Sea Peach* won the MECCA (Montréal English Critics, Circle Award) for Best New Text in 2003. Catherine has performed in Oslo, Bristol and New York, Beijing and Shanghai. Her new book/DVD, *Bipolar Bear,* is available through Conundrum Press. You can contact her at downdogproductions@yahoo.com.

John Malkin is a writer and musician who has been hosting a weekly radio program for seven years on Free Radio Santa Cruz, www.freakradio.org, a commercial-free, collectively run radio station that has been operating without a license from the US government for ten years. John's work has been published in *ascent, Shambhala Sun, Buddhadharma, Z Magazine, In These Times, Alternet, Tricycle Online* and *The Sun.* His book, *Sounds of Freedom,* published by Parallax Press, is a compilation of interviews with musicians speaking about social change and spiritual growth, including Ani DiFranco, the Indigo Girls, Philip Glass, Laurie Anderson and others. John is currently editing a book that highlights

Christian nonviolent peacemakers in America such as Martin Luther King, Jr., Dorothy Day, Thomas Merton and others. He is also working on a book about punk rock and Buddhism, as well as recording music for a CD of original piano music. John Malkin can be reached at jsmalkin@hotmail.com.

Billy Mavreas, Montréal born and based, generally self-identifies as a cartoonist/ comics artist with a tendency toward science fiction/fantasy, psychedelia and "The Occult." His work pivots around the themes of language, sex and perception. Aside from producing a regular strip for *ascent,* he is also a columnist for *Matrix* magazine, is quite active within zinedom and the international mail-art network and also enjoys employing pseudonyms and working anonymously. One can contact him at Monastiraki (the avant garde flea market/art gallery he operates), 5478 Blvd. St. Laurent, Montréal, Quebec, H2T 1S1, Canada. www.yesway.com is his corner of the web.

Marguerite McAfee died on May 26, 2005. In her life, she had been a teacher who worked with children with special needs. She also taught Kundalini Yoga classes until her health no longer permitted it. Through her illness she practised kindness and outstanding compassion. Shortly before Marguerite died, she told a friend that she had overcome her fears and anxiety surrounding her illness. She was strong and ready to move into the unknown.

Michael McColly is currently a lecturer teaching creative nonfiction at Northwestern University. His memoir *Parables of the Body* is published by Soft Skull Press. The memoir blends reportage and interviews as he chronicles his journey through several countries affected by the AIDS epidemic – South Africa, India, Thailand, Vietnam, Senegal and urban America – Chicago. The book focuses on interviews with AIDS activists, NGOs, doctors, social workers, clergy and people like himself who are HIV positive. As he has traveled, he has published journalism, op-ed pieces and essays on the AIDS epidemic in the *New York Times, Salon, Chicago Tribune, The Sun, ascent, The Chronicle of Higher Education,* and other literary journals. He frequently speaks on the international AIDS pandemic at universities and forums in and around Chicago.

Bruce McCoubrey is a realtor for Royal LePage in Vancouver and writes regularly on arts and lifestyle issues. He can be reached at bruce@dreamcityhomes.com.

Clea McDougall was the editor of *ascent* magazine from 1999–2004. She now works as a senior editor for timeless books. She continues to write, edit, and explore the expression of yoga through language, art and life.

Lesley Marian Neilson lives in Victoria, BC with her partner and their twin girls. Her writing mind likes to explore stories about community, ecology, food security and cultural phenomena. She can be contacted at lesley@rocketday.com.

Eileen Delehanty Pearkes lives in the Columbia Mountains of southeastern BC. She is the author of *The Geography of Memory* (a landscape history of the Sinixt First Nation, available through www.sononis.com,) as well as numerous essays that explore the connection between landscape and the human imagination.

Anand Ramayya is a Gemini Award–winning filmmaker and independent producer. He grew up in a film family and has been working on films from the age of fifteen. Anand spent several formative years in his twenties working and backpacking extensively through Asia. Profoundly influenced by his time in Asia, he returned to Canada to pursue a career in film and television. Years later Anand has created a small independent production company committed to producing timely, relevant and challenging international films. See www.kahani.ca for more information.

Gem Salsberg was raised in the wilds throughout Canada and spent many years planting trees across BC and Alberta. Much of her early learning was from her mother's home-schooling, with a focus on exploring nature, creativity and the arts. She has studied art and wilderness exploration at the Atlin Art and Wilderness center, fine arts at the Kootenay School of The Arts and the Emily Carr Institute of Art and Design. Gem is a certified Hatha Yoga teacher, having studied in depth the practice and philosophy of yoga at Yasodhara Ashram. Her writing has also been published in *dANDelion* and her award-winning experimental films have been shown at the Dawson City International Short Film Festival. Gem continues to live her life devoted to the creative poetry that is alive in each moment.

Sparrow lives in Phoenicia, New York, within the Catskill Mountain Range. He is currently studying Hebrew, Buddhism and Duke Ellington. Sparrow's new book is *America: A Prophecy* (Soft Skull Press). sparrow44@juno.com.

Swami Gopalananda has been a long-time student of yoga. He started in 1980 after meeting Swami Sivananda Radha at Yasodhara Ashram in British Columbia. Within two years of their meeting, Swami Gopalananda moved to the ashram with his family, where he has lived ever since. In 1991, he was initiated into *sanyas* by Swami Radha, and today he serves on the ashram's board of directors. Swami Gopalananda is the author of *Can You Listen to a Woman*, an autobiography of his spiritual journey with Swami Radha.

Swami Sivananda (Don Gamble) was the chief of staff and environmental advisor for the World Bank–sponsored independent review of the Sardar Sarovar dam project on the Narmada River. Trained as an environmental engineer in Canada and the United Kingdom, he spent over twenty-five years dealing with the effects of large-scale resource projects, from Arctic oil and gas development and Great Lakes pollution issues in Canada and the United States to this dam mega-project in India. Shortly after the Narmada report was issued in 1992, he moved to Yasodhara Ashram in British Columbia where he now lives, having taking initiation into *sanyas* as Swami Sivananda. He refers to his experience with the people of the Narmada Valley, the government of India and the World Bank as a transformative highlight of his professional career.

Sarah E. Truman spent two years in China researching Guan Yin and studying Qi Gong and Mandarin. She now lives in Canada where she edits *ascent* magazine and is working on a book about Guan Yin to be published in 2007 by timeless books. yueqiuzhen@yahoo.com.

Reverend Ruth Wright has continued in her role at First United and concurrently completed a D.Min. degree at the Vancouver School of Theology. The focus of the project for the degree was the theology of female sex workers. In September 2004, she started a one-year sabbatical during which she toured New Zealand and visited several Mauri ministries, visited Great Britain and France, then spent three months as a volunteer with a mission of the Methodist churches of southern Africa. She is currently trying to digest all she's seen and learned in an effort to take back to First those things that may be of help in their ministry.

resources, bibliographies & websites

Tenzin Palmo Is Watering the Nuns
Tenzin Palmo interviewed by Lesley Marian Neilson
Reflections on a Mountain Lake by Tenzin Palmo (Snow Lion, 2003)
Cave in the Snow by Vicki MacKenzie (Bloomsbury, 1999)
To learn more about Tenzin Palmo's teachings and nunnery visit
www.gatsal.org or www.tenzinpalmo.com

A Day in the Life of Reverend Ruth Wright
by Reverend Ruth Wright
For more information about Vancouver's First United Church,
or how to donate, contact:
First United Church
320 East Hastings Street
Vancouver, V6A 1P4
Ph: (604) 681-8365
Fax: (604) 681-8928

It Takes a Genius To Be Simple: A Profile of Satish Kumar
by Lesley Marian Neilson
Satish Kumar's books include:
The Buddha and the Terrorist: The Story of Angulimala (Green Books, 2005)
You Are, Therefore I Am: A Declaration of Dependence (Green Books, 2002)
Path Without Destination: An Autobiography (William Morrow, 1999)
Resurgence Magazine www.resurgence.org.

The Blessed & Cursed Catastrophe We Call Death & Dying
Joan Halifax Roshi interviewed by Clea McDougall
Joan Halifax Roshi's books include:
A Buddhist Life in America: Simplicity in the Complex (Paulist Press, 1998)
The Fruitful Darkness: Reconnecting With the Body of the Earth (Harper Collins, 1993)
Upaya www.upaya.org

Accident Prone
by Soren Gordhamer
Soren Gordhamer's books include:
Just Say Om!: Your Life's Journey (Adam's Media, 2001)
Meetings With Mentors: A Young Adult Interviews Leading Visionaries
         (Hanford Mead Publishers, 1995)
Lineage Project www.lineageproject.org

Opening to the Unknown
Bo Lozoff interviewed by Soren Gordhamer
Bo Lozoff's books include:
It's a Meaningful Life – It Just Takes Practice (Viking/Penguin, 2001)
We're All Doing Time: A guide for getting free (Human Kindness Foundation, 1984)
www.humankindness.org

Sahodaran
by Micheal McColly
Michael McColly's books include:
Parables of the Body (Soft Skull Press, 2005)
HIV/AIDS resources cited in the article:
Naz Foundation: www.nfi.net
Sahodaran: sahodara@md3.vsnl.net.in
Positive Women Network (PWN+): www.pwnetwork.org
Y.R. Gaitonde Centre for AIDS Research & Education (YRG CARE): www.yrgcare.org

Valley of Tigers
Arundhati Roy interviewed by Swami Sivananda
Books by Arundhati Roy include:

An Ordinary Person's Guide to Empire (South End Press, 2004)
War Talk (South End Press, 2003)
Power Politics (South End Press, 2001)
The Cost of Living (Modern Library, 1999)
The God of Small Things (HarperCollins, 1998)
International Rivers Network www.irn.org
The Friends of the River Narmada www.narmada.org

Theory into Practice
George Feuerstein interviewed by Swami Gopalananda
Books by Georg Feuerstein include:
*The Deeper Dimension of Yoga: Theory and Practice (*Shambhala, 2004*)*
The Shambhala Encyclopedia of Yoga (Shambhala, 2000)
Tantra: The Path of Ecstasy (Shambhala, 1998)
Traditional Yoga Sudies www.yrec.info

Natural Buddha: Meeting Thomas Merton
by Brent Burbridge
Books by Thomas Merton include:
The Seven Story Mountain: 50th Anniversary Edition (Harcourt, 1999)
Mystics and Zen Masters (Farrar, Straus and Giroux, 1999)
The Asian Journal of Thomas Merton (New Directions Publishing, 1975)
Zen and the Birds of Appetite (New Directions Publishing, 1968)

Determined To Be Free
Brother Wayne Teasdale, Thubten Chodron and Swami Radhananda interviewed by
Clea McDougall
Brother Wayne Teasdale's books include:
*Awakening the Spirit, Inspiring the Soul: 30 Stories of Interspiritual Discovery in the
    Community of Faiths* (Deep Books, 2004)
A Monk in the World: Cultivating a Spiritual Life (New World Library, 2002)
The Mystic Heart: Discovering a Universal Spirituality in the World's Religions (New World
    Library, 2001)
Bhikshuni Thubten Chodron's books include:
How to Free Your Mind: Tara the Liberator (Snow Lion Publications, 2005)

Taming the Mind (Snow Lion Publications, 2004)
Buddhism for Beginners (Snow Lion Publications, 2001)
www.thubtenchodron.org or www.sravastiabbey.org.
Swami Radhananda writes a regular column for *ascent* magazine
www.ascentmagazine.com and Yasodhara Ashram www.yasodhara.org

The Ingredients of Love
bell hooks interviewed by Juniper Glass
bell hooks' recent books include:
The Will To Change: Men, Masculinity And Love (Simon and Schuster, 2004)
Rock My Soul: Black People and Self-Esteem (Simon and Schuster, 2004)
Teaching Community: A Pedagogy Of Hope (Routledge, 2003)
All About Love: New Visions (HarperCollins, 2001)

Mary-Jo
by Eileen Delehanty Pearkes
To find out more about Mary-Jo's teaching and projects visit
www.mary-jo.com and www.trinityyoga.com

Fireworks: An Elemental Investigation Sparked by Geeta Iyengar
by Juniper Glass
Geeta Iyengar's books include:
Yoga: A Gem for Women (timeless books, 2005)
Yoga In Action: A Preliminary Course (YOG, 1999)
www.bksiyengar.com

Against the Stream
Noah Levine interviewed by John Malkin
Dharma Punx (HarperCollins, 2004)
www.dharmapunx.com

Kumar
by Jeffry Farrell
Kumar's film roles include:
"Shopkeeper" in *Romance and Cigarettes*, John Turturro/ Humperdink, 2005

"Gupta Rajan, Airport Janitor" in *The Terminal*, Steven Spielberg/Dreamworks, 2004
"Pagoda, The Indian Butler" in *The Royal Tenenbaums*, Wes Anderson/ Disney, 2001
"Mr. Littlejeans, Groundskeeper" in *Rushmore*, Wes Anderson/ Disney, 1998
"Kumar, The Safecracker" in *Bottle Rocket*, Wes Anderson/ Columbia, 1996
www.kumarpallana.com, www.theamazingkumar.com

Blemish
David Sylvian interviewed by Marcus Boon
David Sylvian's CDs include:
The Good Son vs. The Only Daughter (Samadhi Sound, 2005)
World Citizen (Samadhi Sound, 2004)
Blemish (Samadhi Sound, 2003)
Dead Bees on a Cake (Virgin, 1999)
Secrets of the Beehive (Virgin, 1987)
Brilliant Trees (Virgin, 1984)
Tin Drum (as Japan) (Caroline, 1981)
www.samadhisound.com

Adrift with Yann Martel
Yann Martel interviewed by Bruce McCobrey
Yann Martel's books include:
Life of Pi (Knopf Vintage Canada, 2002)
Facts Behind the Helsinki Roccamatios (Vintage Canada, 2002)
Self (Vintage Canada, 1993)

A Cosmic Current
by Anand Ramayya
Based on the film *Cosmic Current*, Anand Ramayya, produced by Joe MacDonald, 2004
www.kahani.ca

information on ascent magazine, timeless books & yasodhara ashram

ascent magazine

To subscribe to or order back issues of *ascent* magazine contact:

837 rue Gilford

Montréal, QC H2J 1P1

Canada

Toll free: 1-888-825-0228

info@ascentmagazine.com

www.ascentmagazine.com

timeless books

timeless titles by Swami Sivananda Radha:

Mantras: Words of Power

Hatha Yoga: The Hidden Language

The Devi of Speech: The Goddess in Kundalini Yoga

When You First Called Me Radha: Poems

Kundalini Yoga for the West

Realities of the Dreaming Mind

Radha: Diary of a Woman's Search

for a free timeless catalogue or more info:

Canada toll free: 1-800-661-8711

USA toll free: 1-800-251-9273

contact@timeless.org

www.timeless.org

The Yasodhara Ashram

If you would like to make a donation to either timeless books or *ascent* magazine, or for information on courses and retreats at Yasodhara Ashram, contact:

Toll free: 1-800-661-8711

yashram@netidea.com

www.yasodhara.org